100 HEALTHY BODY ACTIVITIES FOR KIDS IDEAS IN 2022

NICHOLAS NEHLS

Annotation

Yoga can solve absolutely all health problems, tipichnye for modern children. Yoga is not a sport. changes, proidescending in a person practicing yoga, affect not only him body,but his mind, and soul, and all these changes are only for the better. Atyoga classes do not require any special equipment, dorogoy clothes, a separate room. For daily workouts needbut only a well-ventilated room, a thin rug (or blanket) and easyth, non-restrictive sports suit. And, of course, desireand good mood.

Yoga. Introduction for children

The word "yoga" comes from the word "yoj" ("yuj"), which in translation from the ancient Sanskrit language sounds like "connection", "connection", "union". This name speaks for itself - the essence of yoga philosophy is to achieve a merger, an inextricable connection between the human Soul and the Highest Divine Will.

In other words, yoga helps a person to realize himself as a particle of the big world and to feel his close connection with all living things.

Yoga classes are not only exercises for the body, but also for the spirit. By mastering yoga exercises, a person not only strengthens his physical health, but also learns internal discipline, control over his emotions, the ability to relax and rest not only with his body, but also with his soul.

Gradually, people practicing yoga give up bad thoughts, words and deeds that cause irreparable harm to the human soul, acquire the ability to distinguish important events from those not worthy of attention, do not get upset over trifles and do not quarrel with other people. All this helps a person learn to live in a state of balance, harmony with himself and with the whole world.

Yoga is a very ancient spiritual teaching that originated over 2,000 years ago. The founder of yoga is the sage Patanjali, who lived in ancient India.

Most of the exercises in yoga - they are called asanas - got their names from the names of animals. In ancient times, people paid attention to the fact that the postures that some animals take can also benefit the human body. For example, stretching like a cat, or bending like a snake, a person performs a real exercise for his spine. That is why these poses got their names "Cat Pose" or "Snake Pose".

You will also get acquainted with asanas named after the ancient legendary heroes and sages of India, or mythical characters - the Fish God Matsindra, the Lord of the Birds Garuda, the God of War Shanmukhi and many others.

In Europe, America and Russia, yoga appeared only at the end of the 20th century. Beautiful postures and the famous calmness, equanimity of yogis aroused great interest, and many people began to get acquainted with this teaching and practice the exercises. Over time, people realized that

Regular yoga practice is good for health andjoy.

General Guidelines Introduction for Parents

Why do kids do yoga?

Disappointing facts about children's health

It is unlikely that anyone would think to challenge the fact that regular physical activity is necessary for every child.

And if someone had thought of this, then it would have been very easy to end the dispute - it would be enough to go to any school and carefully look at the students of the lower and middle classes (there is nothing to say about the older ones).

It's no secret that the health of modern children leaves much to be desired.the best. You can blame bad ecology, heredity, anything, but, as ruthless statistics show, children acquire most health problems, usually at preschool and primary school age.

Poor posture, flat feet, problems with coordination of movements, visual impairment, poor functioning of the digestive system, obesity, inability to concentrate and poor memory - all these problems can be avoided if you pay attention to the child's lifestyle in time.

But all these disorders are not so harmless - a slight stoop by adolescence easily turns into scoliosis, leads to pain in the cervical spine and head, contributes to visual impairment, disrupts the proper functioning of the respiratory system. In an inseparable bundle with the curvature of the spine, flat feet also walk.

Malfunctions in the work of the stomach and intestines are future gastritis, colitis, dysbacteriosis and all their unpleasant consequences - a decrease in immunity, the development of allergic reactions and other autoimmune diseases.

Excess weight not only harms the health of the child (and in the future - and adult), but also causes ridicule from peers.

Inability to concentrate, problems with memory - all this causes difficulties in mastering educational material, and yet the load on the children's brain only grows with each grade of school.

And the value of good vision for each person can not be mentioned.

The saddest thing is that in most cases all these problems have two roots - malnutrition and lack of movement.

Physical inactivity is one of the biggest problems of the modern world, in which a person has practically lost the urgent need for movement, and with it his health.

It is she who "gives" us extra pounds, weakens our heart and blood vessels, makes our intestines lazy, deprives our organs of vital oxygen, stoops our backs ...

And, unfortunately, all these problems are unstoppable every year.

"getting younger". Children sit for hours at lessons - at school and at home - with hunched backs; "rest" on the couch in front of the TV, or curled up in front of the computer; the time of active promotion of sports and children's activities in free sports sections, unfortunately, has passed; there are fewer and fewer people who want to play football on the street ...

The lack of habit of movement gives rise to laziness and a desire to move as little as possible, it is already difficult to force atrophied muscles to do some work, a simple climb up the stairs is perceived as hard work and requires a long rest - a vicious circle is obtained.

And your child falls into this circle. Think about it!

And after all, only we, adults, in whose power to give children a happy healthy life, can break this circle, we can acquaint the child with the joy of movement and direct him along the right path.

Whyexactly yoga?

Why more and more parents around the world, choosing the type of physical activity for their children, prefer yoga? After all, there are many sports.

The answer is simple: because yoga is not a sport. The changes that occur in a person practicing yoga affect not only his body, but also his mind and soul, and all these changes are only for the better.

If we talk about the physical aspect of yoga, then this type of activity should be preferred, if only because in it, unlike most sports, injuries are practically impossible. All movements in yoga are smooth and unhurried, and performing exercises according to exact recommendations, it is simply impossible to harm your body.

Children who have suffered damage to the spine, brain, joints, suffering from chronic diseases, should

start yoga classes only after consulting a doctor and an experienced instructor. Only they will be able to give competent advice on the correct selection of asanas and the timing of their implementation.

Meanwhile, it is yoga that allows you to solve absolutely all health problems typical of modern children.

Most of the exercises in yoga in one way or another affect the spine. All stretching and twisting of the spinal column not only increase its flexibility, improve the nutrition of each vertebra, contribute to the formation and maintenance of correct posture, but also allow you to compensate for the negative impact of incorrect, non-physiological postures in which the child finds himself during the day.

Strengthening the muscles of the back and abdomen provides the spine with reliable support.

The development of mobility of the cervical spine improves brain nutrition, relieves eye strain, and helps improve the ability to concentrate, understand and assimilate new information. Moreover, neck exercises are very useful for children suffering from frequent colds affecting the throat and nasopharynx.

The expansion of the chest, which occurs during the performance of many asanas, helps the lungs to open in full, eliminates disturbances in the functioning of the respiratory system and relieves chronic bronchopulmonary diseases. These exercises also improve the functioning of the cardiovascular system.

During most of the yoga exercises, all the organs of the abdominal cavity experience a gentle effect, which is often called "internal massage". Improving blood circulation in all internal organs normalizes their work and accelerates the removal of decay products, toxins and toxins from the body. Especially importantstimulation of intestinal peristalsis - it is precisely its violation, the accumulation of toxic substances in the body that lead to the development of a huge number of diseases.

Proper functioning of all internal organs normalizes metabolic processes, improves the absorption of all nutrients from food. Children who practice yoga gradually normalize their weight - lean children become more dense, and those who are overweight get rid of body fat. This moment is especially important for adolescents during a period of rapid growth and hormonal changes in the body.

All yoga exercises contribute to the development of certain muscles.

Of course, yogis are not like bodybuilders, but their physical form is the form of a beautiful and healthy person.

Regular practice of asanas has a positive effect on the psyche of the child. Scattered children become more collected, while those who suffer from a lack of attention learn to concentrate. Yoga also helps to cope with hyperactivity, the problem of many modern children. Smooth slow movements, immobility in postures, relaxation - all these features of yoga exercises make children calmer and allow them to get rid of not only physical, but also emotional stress.

Yoga has another indisputable advantage over many sports - yoga does not require any special equipment, expensive clothes, a separate room. For daily workouts, all you need is a well-ventilated room, a thin mat (or blanket), and a light, non-restrictive tracksuit. Well, and, of course, desire and good mood.

Boys andgirls

Other parents may say: developed muscles and endurance, which appears with a long stay in yoga asanas, the ability to cope with one's emotions - all this is very useful for boys, but is it really necessary for girls?

Certainly, it is necessary.

The development of correct posture, easy gait, the appearance of smoothness and grace in movements - all this is much more important for growing girls than ideal forms.

Yes, and figure defects are quite amenable to correction with the help of asanas.

- the legs become more slender, the buttocks are tightened, the stomach is flat, the chest is raised.

And, undoubtedly, girls will appreciate how clean and smooth the skin of the face will become due to the normalization of the functioning of the gastrointestinal tract.

The growing girl develops harmoniously, turning into a beautiful, self-confident girl. Isn't that what every loving parent wants for their daughter?

Moreover, there are some aspects of the influence of yoga specifically onfemale body. Exercises that move the pelvis normalize blood circulation in this area, and this is the best prevention of many gynecological diseases.

Good functioning of the reproductive organs, developed and elastic

muscles in the future make such a girl more prepared for bearing and giving birth to a healthy child.

The practice of yoga in the period preceding menstruation helps the girl cope with irritability and tension, which are not uncommon at this time, and a number of asanas alleviate discomfort during the period itself.

"critical days"

Yoga classes for children of all ages

Classes with preschoolers and younger students

Younger children, of course, will need your help during classes. If you practice yoga yourself, then it will not be difficult for you to master asanas with your child. If you are just starting to get acquainted with this ancient philosophy of health and harmony, then you will first need to carefully study all the recommendations given in this book yourself.

Look at the photos attached to each exercise, read the description of the asana and try it yourself. It does not matter if at first you cannot reach the floor with your hand or throw your legs over your head - perhaps your baby will cope with this better, because children are more flexible.

However, keep in mind that there is nothing more stimulating for children than the example of their parents. Therefore, do not refuse the opportunity to discover the world of yoga for yourself. It will only benefit you.

Having analyzed all the exercises of the complex, try to remember the sequence of movements as best as possible - after all, you will become the first yoga teacher for your child.

When practicing with young children, do not invite them to memorize the Indian names of asanas - name the exercises using the Russian translation: "Locust Pose", "Dog Pose", "Lion Pose". Children are usually fascinated by this "animal game", and they quickly remember the correct position of the body.

It is possible to introduce children to asanas from a very young age.

- from 2-3 years old, as soon as the child can remember the names of animals. Use large color pictures and offer your child

"stretch like a cat", "sit like a frog", "stand like a tree".

Of course, these play sessions will not be yoga classes in the full sense, but they will gradually prepare the child for the exercises that you will do with him in the future.

With children from 4–5 years old, you can engage in using already wholesets of exercises. However, do not turn these activities into physical education.

- do not turn away from pictures and toys that help the child "enter into

image", come up with a short story about a merry journey of some fabulous creature, meeting various animals on its way, turning either into a mountain or into a tree. The need to freeze for a few seconds in the asana is explained by magical charms.

Do not forget to praise the child every time and rejoice at his success.Activities with teenagers

Children from 10-12 years old can do yoga on their own, but they may still need your advice or help.

Teenagers, unlike kids, are very attracted to the classic names of exercises, so each of them is offered in a book with translations of all the words of which it consists. Stimulate your child's cognitive activity - invite him to learn more about mythological characters and legendary heroes, whose names formed the basis for the names of certain asanas. This knowledge will fill children's yoga classes with deep meaning.

At this age, children are already able to concentrate on their own feelings, so pay your child's attention to moments of tension and relaxation of certain muscle groups, encourage him to monitor his breathing, adhering to the recommendations given in the book.

Pay attention to the child that during his stay in the asana he should try to arouse pleasant thoughts in himself.

Control the speed at which your child masters certain exercises

- gently stimulate him to develop his flexibility and endurance, increasing the time spent in the asana and the accuracy of the exercise, but do not force events - each organism has its own capabilities.

Recommendations for classes

Remember, in order for yoga to give the best result, you need to start your acquaintance with it in a good mood, with faith in your own strength, with a calm and friendly attitude towards the world around you.

Then everything will definitely work out! Place for yoga

To perform all the exercises, you will definitely need a hard, flat surface. It is best to start classes on the floor, laying a thin rug (you can use a tourist one) or a thin blanket on it. Pay attention to the fact that the rug does not slip under your feet. Keep your carpet clean.

Practice yoga in a room that is well ventilated. The temperature in the practice room should be at least 17-18 ° C if you are exercising in a tracksuit. Those who prefer light T-shirts and shorts need a warmer room. The main rule: you should be comfortable - neither hot nor cold, fresh enough, but without drafts. Performing classic yoga asanas involves barefoot, and your feet should not freeze - this will distract you, interfere with concentration on the accepted position.

It's good if you have the opportunity to practice in front of a large mirror - this way you can better control the correctness of the exercise. In any case, when starting to master asanas, do it only with open eyes.

In summer, you can also practice outdoors - laying a rug on the ground or sand. Choose shady places where you will not be disturbed by insects.

Time for yoga

It's great if you can start every morning with yoga exercises. So your body can gently wake up, and you will get a boost of energy for the whole day.

However, you can practice in the daytime or in the evening, but not earlier than 3 hours after eating. Of course, this is not always easy, and 1-2 hours before the start of classes, you can drink a cup of tea, milk, cocoa.

In the summer, do not do yoga if you have spent several hours in the bright sun - stay in the shade for 30-40 minutes, relax.

Before starting a lesson, you should, if possible, empty your intestines and bladder, blow your nose thoroughly, and take a shower. After finishing your exercise, rest for 10-15 minutes before heading to the shower.

You should do it every day - at least - at least 5-6 times a week.

In the first weeks, the duration of your classes will be no more than 15-20 minutes, gradually you will increase it to 45 minutes. The daily set of exercises can be divided into two blocks and performed one in the morning, and the second in the afternoon or evening.

If classes are led by parents, then they should select a group of more active, stimulating exercises from the complex and offer them in the morning, and leave simpler, calming and relaxing exercises for the evening.

Of course, it is not forbidden to perform yoga asanas in the interval between classes: if you are tired from sitting for a long time, they will help you stretch your muscles and improve blood circulation in the body, if, on the contrary, you are physically tired, asanas will help get rid of muscle tension and give your body rest .

However, it should be remembered that yoga should not cause overwork. After physical activity, perform only those exercises that make you feel relaxed, you should start more intense asanas only after having a good rest.

Master new exercises gradually, gradually increasing the load, carefully preparing your body for each new asana. Remember: there is no single pace for mastering yoga exercises for everyone - each person is individual, and, depending on his physical form and state of health, certain poses will be easy for him or cause difficulties.

If you lead an active lifestyle, go in for sports, then it is best to organize your day so that there is a gap between your classes, at least 4-5 hours.

Clothing for classesyoga

The main requirement for clothing for classes is that it should be loose enough so that you can easily take any, the most intricate pose. The ability of the fabric to pass air is also important - your clothes should "breathe" and not interfere with your skin's breathing. Therefore, give preference to things made from natural fabrics - cotton and linen. You don't need shoes or socks to practice yoga.

Contraindications for yoga

In no case do not exercise if you have a fever or a cold in full swing. Many asanas are very useful for speeding up recovery in various acute respiratory infections and acute respiratory infections, but they are best used at the stage of recovery.

With caution, you need to start training for those who have a tendency to increase blood pressure, and for children suffering from chronic diseases. In these cases, you must first consult with your doctor.

Girls on "critical days", even if their condition is generally quite satisfactory, should moderate their activity. All "inverted poses" (Sarvangasana, Halasana), any asanas associated with strong compression or stretching of the pelvis and abdomen (Hanumasana), standing and sitting poses can be performed with support and support (for example, in the Lion Pose, lower the buttocks without on the floor, but on a rolled-up blanket).

But before the start of a new cycle (during PMS), poses with inclinations, asanas in the prone position, deep and calm breathing help relieve mental stress.

Mastering asanas

Recommendations for the selection of the complex

It takes 1-2 weeks to master each set of asanas. It is clear that the first sets of exercises - the simplest ones - can be mastered faster than subsequent complicated ones.

Mastering the exercise for the first time, do it once or twice, as accurately as possible. The next day, add one to two repetitions, trying to increase the time spent in the asana by at least a few seconds. Bring the number of repetitions to 5-10 times.

Having met an already mastered exercise in the next complex, perform it 5 times during the week, gradually increasing the time spent in the asana.

In the future, when performing the same exercises, be guided by the degree of its development, your well-being and the amount of free time. Gradually, you can reduce the number of repetitions of simple exercises to 1-2 times, increasing the time spent in the asana and the number of exercises performed.

If you have not fully mastered any exercise from the previous complex, then add it to the next complex, even if it was not originally included in it.

Below are the various sets of asanas.

Each complex is divided into two parts: the first includes 5-6 exercises, which must be completed. From the second part, choose exercises at your discretion, trying to perform different types of asanas, for example, one - sitting, the second - lying on your stomach, the third - lying on your back.

Number of exercises from the second partdepends on the age of the child - it is quite enough for young children to add 2-3 exercises to the main complex, and teenagers can perform 5-6 or even more.

You can set aside extra time to complete thoseexercises that help you solve a specific problem

develop a sense of balance, form a good posture, develop the muscles of any group, etc. Having mastered all the complexes proposed in the book, you can create several of your own using the mastered exercises.

When compiling complexes, arrange the asanas in the following order:

i.   standing exercises

v.   lying exercises

v.   sitting exercises Complexes of asanas Complex 1 First part

Tadasana (Samasthiti) - Mountain Pose Vrikshasana - Tree Pose

Utthita Trikonasana - Stretched Triangle PoseUtthita Parshvakonasana - Extended Side Angle Pose Virabhadrasana I - Warrior Pose I

The second part

Parshvottanasana - Intense Lateral Stretch Pose Salamba Sarvagasana I - Supported Candle Pose I

Halasana - Plow Pose

Maha Mudra– Great Seal

Parivritta Parshvakonasana – Twisted Side Angle Pose Complex 2

First part

Tadasana (Samasthiti) - Mountain Pose Vrikshasana - Tree Pose

Parivritta Trikonasana -Inverted Triangle PoseParivritta Parshvakonasana - Twisted Side Angle Pose Virabhadrasana I - Warrior Pose I

Virabhadrasana II - Warrior Pose II

The second part

Natarajasana - PoseGod of the Dance

Parshvottanasana - Intense Lateral Stretch Pose Salamba Sarvagasana I - Supported Candle Pose I

Halasana - Plow Pose Virasana - Hero PoseBakasana – Crane Pose Complex 3

First part

Utthita Trikonasana - Stretched Triangle PoseUtthita Parshvakonasana - Extended Side Angle Pose Virabhadrasana I - Warrior Pose I

VirabhadrasanaII – Warrior Pose II Virabhadrasana III – Warrior Pose III

The second part

Natarajasana - PoseGod of the Dance

Salamba Sarvagasana I – Supported Candle Pose I Halasana – Plow Pose

Karnapidasana - Knees to Ears Pose Simhasana I - Lion Pose

Marichiasana III - Sage PoseMarichi III Marichiasana IV - Sage Pose Marichi IV Complex 4

First part

Utthita Trikonasana - Stretched Triangle PoseUtthita Parshvakonasana - Extended Side Angle Pose Virabhadrasana I - Warrior Pose I

Natarajasana - Dance God Pose Ardha Chandrasana - Crescent Moon Pose

The second part

Parshvottanasana - Intense Lateral Stretch Pose Prasarita Padottanasana I - Stretched Foot Pose I Urdhva Prasarita Padanasana - Upward Stretched Feet Pose Rajakapotasana - King Pigeon Pose

Ardha Navasana - Half Boat Pose

Gomukasana (Gomukhasana) - Cow Head Pose Padmasana - Lotus Pose

Complex 5

First part

Utthita Trikonasana - Stretched Triangle PoseParivritta Trikonasana - Inverted Triangle Pose Virabhadrasana III - Warrior Pose III

Ardha Chandrasana - Half Moon Pose

Prasarita Padottanasana I - Stretched Foot Pose I Prasarita Padottanasana II - Stretched Foot Pose II

The second part

Parighasana - Bolt PoseParipurna Navasana - Boat Pose

Rajakapotasana - Pose of the King of PigeonsGomukasana (Gomukhasana) - Cow Head Pose Bakasana - Crane Pose

Padmasana - Lotus Pose Complex 6

First part

Utthita Parsvakonasana - Extended Side Angle Pose Parivritta Parsvakonasana - Twisted Side Angle Pose Padangushthasana - Standing Pose With Thumb GrabPadahastasana–Maximum Stretch Pose Rear

Leg Surfaces

Uttanasana - Intense Spine Stretch Pose

The second part

Urdhva Prasarita Padanasana - Upward Stretched Feet Pose Salamba Sarvangasana I - Supported Candle Pose I

Halasana - Plow Pose

Karnapidasana - PoseKnees to Ears

Eka Pada Sarvangasana - a variation of Sarvangasana, Candle Pose with One Leg Behind the Head

Jathara Parivartanasana - Belly Rotation Pose Dhanurasana - Bow Pose

Urdhva Dhanurasana I - Inverted PoseLuke

Eka Pada Urdhva Dhanurasana – Reverse Bow Pose with Leg Raised Up

Complex 7

First part

Utthita Trikonasana - Extended Triangle Pose Parivrtta Trikonasana - Inverted Triangle Pose Utthita Parshvakonasana - Extended Side Angle PoseParivritta Parshvakonasana – Twisted Side Angle Pose

Natarajasana - PoseGod of the Dance

The second part

Prasarita Padottanasana I – Stretched Foot Pose IPrasarita Padottanasana II – Stretched Foot Pose II

Padangushthasana - Standing Pose with Grab the Big ToesPadahastasana–Maximum Stretch Pose Rear

Leg Surfaces

Uttanasana - Intense Spine Stretch Pose Parighasana - Bolt Posture

Makarasana - Crocodile Pose Dhanurasana - Bow Pose

Urdhva Dhanurasana I - Inverted PoseLuke

Eka Pada Urdhva Dhanurasana – Reverse Bow Pose with Leg Raised Up

Bhujangasana - PoseCobra

Urdhva Prasarita Padanasana - Upward Stretched Feet Pose Paripurna Navasana - Boat Pose

Ardha Navasana - Half Boat Pose

Salamba SarvangasanaI - Supported Candle Pose I Halasana - Plow Pose

Karnapidasana - PoseKnees to Ears

Eka Pada Sarvangasana - a variation of Sarvangasana, Candle Pose with One Leg Behind the Head

Parshvaika Pada Sarvangasana – Pose Candles One foot,Laid aside

Jathara Parivartanasana - Belly Rotation Pose

Setu Bandha Sarvangasana (Uttana Mayurasana) – Bridge Construction Pose

Supta Trivikramasana - Bent Pose Trivikrama Bhujangasana II - Snake Pose II

Marichiasana III - Sage PoseMarichi III Marichiasana IV - Sage Pose Marichi IV Complex 8

First part

Vrikshasana - Tree Pose Virabhadrasana I - Warrior Pose I Virabhadrasana II - Warrior Pose II Virabhadrasana III - Warrior Pose III Natarajasana - Dance God Pose

Parshvottanasana - Intense Lateral Stretch Pose

The second part

Ushtrasana - Camel Pose Utkatasana - Power Pose

Salamba SarvangasanaI - Supported Candle Pose I Halasana - Plow Pose

Karnapidasana - PoseKnees to Ears

Pindasana in Sarvangasana - Fetal Pose inCandle Pose Jathara Parivartanasana - Belly Rotation Pose

Setu Bandha Sarvangasana (Uttana Mayurasana) – Bridge Construction Pose

Bhujangasana II - Snake PoseRajakapotasana - Pose of the King of Pigeons Maha Mudra - Great Seal

Janu Shirshasana - Head Knee PoseChaturanga Dandasana - Staff Pose

Pashchimottanasana (Ugrasana, Brahmacharyasana) – Back and Buttocks Stretch Pose

Chaturanga Dandasana - Staff Pose Kapotasana - Pigeon Pose

Pashchimottanasana (Ugrasana, Brahmacharyasana) – Back and Buttocks Stretch Pose

Rajakapotasana - Pose of the King of Pigeons

Eka Pada RajakapotasanaII - Pose of the King of Pigeons II Complex 9

First part

Utthita Trikonasana - Extended Triangle Pose Parivrtta Trikonasana - Inverted Triangle Pose Utthita Parshvakonasana - Extended Side Angle PoseParivritta Parshvakonasana - Twisted Side Angle Pose Virabhadrasana I - Warrior Pose I

Virabhadrasana II - Warrior Pose II

The second part

Virabhadrasana III -Warrior Pose III Ardha Chandrasana – Crescent Moon Pose

Parshvottanasana - Intense Lateral Stretch Pose Prasarita Padottanasana I - Stretched Foot Pose I Prasarita Padottanasana I - Stretched Foot Pose II

Padangushthasana - Standing Thumb Hold Pose Uttanasana - Intense Spinal Stretch Pose

Urdhva Prasarita Ekapadasana – Reclining Pose with Leg Raised Up

Utkatasana - Power Pose Ushtrasana - Camel PoseShalabhasana - Locust
Pose Dhanurasana - Bow Pose

Chaturanga Dandasana - Staff Pose Bhujangasana - Cobra Pose

Adho muksha (mukha) svanasana - Dog Muzzle PoseDownward Virasana –
Hero Pose

Salamba SarvangasanaI - Supported Candle Pose I Halasana - Plow Pose

Karnapidasana - PoseKnees to Ears

Supta Konasana -Recumbent Angle Pose

Parshva Halasana - Plow Pose with Legs Behind Head

Eka Pada Sarvangasana - a variation of Sarvangasana, Candle Pose with
One Leg Behind the Head

Jathara Parivartanasana - Belly Rotation Pose Chakrasana - Wheel Pose

Janu Shirshasana - Head Knee PoseParivrtta Janu Shirshasana

Maha Mudra - Great SealChaturanga Dandasana - Staff Pose

Purvottanasana - Inverted Plank Eastern Stretch Pose Eka Pada
Rajakapotasana II - King of Pigeons Pose II

Eka Pada Rajakapotasana IV – PoseKing of Pigeons IV Hanumasana –
Monkey King Pose

Complex 10

First part

Salamba SarvangasanaI - Supported Candle Pose I Halasana - Plow Pose

Karnapidasana - Knees to Ears Pose Supta Konasana - Reclining Angle Pose

Parshva Halasana - Plow Pose with Legs Behind Head

Eka Pada Sarvangasana - a variation of Sarvangasana, Candle Pose with
One Leg Behind the Head

The second part

ParshvaikaPadaSarvangasana–ProseCandlesOne foot,Laid aside

Jathara Parivartanasana - Belly Rotation Pose Chakrasana - Wheel Pose

Paripurna Navasana - Boat Pose Ardha Navasana - Half Boat
PoseChaturanga Dandasana - Staff Pose Bhujangasana - Cobra Pose

Maha Mudra– Great Seal

Janu Shirshasana - Head Knee PoseTriang Mukhai Kapada Pashchi
Mottanasana Ardha Baddha Padma Pashchimottanasana Marichiasana I –
Sage Marichi Pose I Marichiasana II – Sage Marichi Pose II Upavistha
Konasana – Seated Angle Pose

Parivritta Paschimottanasana – Reverse Pose Back and Buttocks Stretches

Urdhva Mukha Pashchimottanasana I - Facing Back Stretch I

Purvottanasana - Inverted Plank Pose Eastern Stretch Bharadvajasana I -
Bharadvaja I Pose

Bharadvajasana II - Bharadwaja II Pose Malasana I - Garland Pose I

Malasana II - Garland Pose IIBaddha Konasana - Butterfly Pose Padmasana
- Lotus Pose

Shanmukhi Mudra - Sealing Pose Simhasana - Lion Pose

VamadevasanaI - Sage Vamadeva Pose I

Eka Pada Rajakapotasana II - Pose of the King of Pigeons II Eka Pada Rajakapotasana IV - Pose of the King of Pigeons IV Hanumasana - Pose of the King of Monkeys

Samakonasana - Right Angle Pose Complex 11

First part

Utkatasana– Power Pose

Padangushthasana - Standing Thumb Hold Pose Ardha Baddha Padmottanasana - Standing Half Lotus Pose

leg

Garudasana - Eagle PoseVatayanasana - Horse Pose

Salamba Sarvangasana I – Supported Candle Pose I

The second part

Halasana - Plow Pose

Karnapidasana - Knees to Ears Pose Supta Konasana - Reclining Angle Pose

Parshva Halasana - Plow Pose with Legs Behind Head

Eka Pada Sarvangasana - a variation of Sarvangasana, Candle Pose with One Leg Behind the Head

ParshvaikaPadaSarvangasana–ProseCandlesOne foot,Laid aside

Jathara Parivartanasana - Belly Rotation PoseUrdhva Prasarita Padasana - Upward Stretched Feet Pose Anantasana - Ananta Serpent Back Pose

Supta Padangushthasana – Thumb Leg Stretch Pose in Lying Position

Urdhva Mukha Pashchimottanasana II - Back Stretch Facing II

Shalabhasana - Locust Pose Dhanurasana - Bow Pose

Parshva Dhanurasana - PoseBow on Side Matsyasana - Fish Pose

Padangushta Dhanurasana Supta Virasana - Hero Bhakasana Pose

Simhasana - Lion Pose

Siddhasana - Perfect Pose (Sage Pose) Triang Mukhai Kapada Pashchi Mottanasana Kraunchasana - Heron Pose

Vamadevasana I - Sage Vamadeva PoseI Hanumasana - Monkey King Pose Samakonasana - Right Angle Pose Kurmasana - Turtle Pose

Complex 12

First part

Utthita Trikonasana - Extended Triangle Pose Parivrtta Trikonasana - Inverted Triangle Pose Utthita Parshvakonasana - Extended Side Angle PoseParivritta Parshvakonasana - Twisted Side Angle Pose Ardha Chandrasana - Crescent Moon Pose

Utthita Hasta Padangushthasana - Hand and Big Toe Pose

The second part

Parighasana - Bolt Pose Ushtrasana - Camel Pose Garudasana - Eagle PoseShalabhasana - Locust Pose

Adho muksha (mukha) svanasana - Dog Muzzle PoseDownward Anantasana - Ananta Serpent Back Pose

Uttana padasana - Raise Arms and Legs Pose

Setu Bandha Sarvangasana (Uttana Mayurasana) – Bridge Construction Pose

Salamba Sarvangasana I – Supported Candle Pose I

Halasana - Plow Pose

Karnapidasana - Knees to Ears PoseGomukasana (Gomukhasana) - Cow Head Pose Simhasana - Lion Pose

Baddha Konasana - Butterfly Pose Matsyasana - Fish Pose

Baddha Padmasana - Closed Lotus Pose Supta Vajrasana - Sleeping Lightning Pose Yoga Mudrasana - Yoga Seal

Marichiasana I - Sage Marichi Pose I Marichiasana II - Sage Marichi Pose II Crownchasana - Heron Pose

Malasana I - Garland Pose I

Ardha Matsyendrasana - Half Matsyendra Pose (Matsyendra - Fish God)

Pashasana - Loop PoseKurmasana - Turtle Pose

Supta Kurmasana - Sleeping Turtle Pose Complex 13

First part

Natarajasana - PoseGod of the Dance

Utthita Hasta Padangushthasana - Hand and Big Toe Pose

Urdhva Prasarita Ekapadasana – Reclining Pose with Leg Raised Up

Bhekasana (Mandukasana) - Frog Pose

Urdhva Mukha Pashchimottanasana II - Back Stretch Facing II

The second part

Akarna Dhanurasana - PoseArcher

Salamba Sarvangasana I – Supported Candle Pose I

Eka Pada Sarvangasana - a variation of Sarvangasana, Candle Pose with
One Leg Behind the Head

ParshvaikaPadaSarvangasana–ProseCandlesOne foot,Laid aside

Setu Bandha Sarvangasana (Uttana Mayurasana) – Bridge Construction
Pose

Padangushtha Dhanurasana - Bow Pose with Thumb Hold

Nog

Bhekasana (Mandukasana) - PoseFrogs Vamadevasana I - Sage Vamadeva I
Hanumasana - Monkey King Pose Samakonasana - Right Angle
PoseUpavistha Konasana - Seated Angle Pose Kurmasana - Turtle Pose

Supta Kurmasana - Sleeping Turtle Pose Malasana I - Garland Pose I

Bakasana - Crane PoseKapotasana - Dove Pose

Eka Pada Galavasana - Sage PoseGalavas with One Leg Supta Bhekasana –
Inverted Frog Pose

Dwi Pada Viparita Dandasana – Reversed Staff Pose Tips

If you can't immediately complete any exercise correctly, don't be discouraged. Yoga is not a sport, there are no competitions and race for the championship. Gradually, with the development of flexibility, as a result of regular practice, you will be able to master the most difficult asanas.

At the initial stage, do the exercise as best as you can, each time trying to make it a little better, to stay in the asana a little longer. Remember that even an asana performed "half-heartedly" has a positive effect on the body. But, of course, this is not a reason not to try to perform the exercise perfectly.

It is best to postpone an exercise that causes you discomfort for 1-2 weeks, and then return to it.

Most difficult asanas have easier options (for example, Locust Pose and Half Locust Pose). Start your acquaintance with yoga poses with simpler exercises and, when they become easy for you, move on to more complex ones.

The main health problems of modern people include problems with the spine. Therefore, pay special attention to those postures that develop the flexibility and mobility of the spinal column, strengthen the back muscles, and help form the correct posture.

All postures in which the load on the body is distributed asymmetrically

- for example, when stretching one leg, when turning or tilting to one side - it must be done for each side.

To make it easier for you to do bending poses, perform each bending on the exhale after a deep breath.

Breathing while performing asanas is only necessarynose!

A whole section is devoted to breath control in yoga - pranayama, but it is difficult for young children to control their breathing, so you only need to make sure that when doing all the exercises, the child breathes evenly and calmly, without delay.

Perform all exercises smoothly, without making sudden movements. Before starting the exercise, try to relax all your muscles - this way you will make them more flexible, plastic.

As you master each new pose, pay attention to the order of actions that guarantees you the best result:

1. Relaxation

Performing each exercisestart with rest and relaxation. Sit or lie down so that you can relax all your muscles. Take 3 deep breaths and exhale.

2. Asana setup

Take a good look at the photos of the asana and carefully read the description of the exercise. Mentally imagine all the changes in body position, step by step.

3. Entryin asana

Perform all movements in the sequence indicatedin the exercise description. Move from one movement to another smoothly, slowly. Do not force the exercise - a little pain when stretching the muscles is quite normal, but you should not experience severe discomfort.

4. Residencein asana

Having taken the final position of the asana, one should linger in it.

When mastering the pose, linger in it for no more than 5 seconds. If it is easy for you, every day increase the time spent in it by 1-2 seconds, no more. If being in an asana causes you difficulty, then increase the time every few days.

For children under 12 years old, it is quite enough to bring the time spent in the asana to 10-20 seconds. Older children can increase this time to 1-3 minutes.

Think about something pleasant at this time.

5. Exit from the asana

Very slowly and smoothly reverse all movements and return to the starting position.

6. Relaxation

After doing any exercise, relax while sitting or lying down.

Rest time should be at least half the time spent on the exercise.

After completing the complex, rest, relaxing with your eyes closed, for a few minutes. In this case, the rest time should not be less than the time spent on the implementation of the complex.

Preparing to perform asanas

Even if you regularlyyou play sports, you have a good stretch and developed muscles, before you start mastering asanas, you need a little warm-up.

Warm-up, complexone

1. Stand on the floor with your back pressed against the wall with your heels, shins, buttocks, shoulders and back of your head. Count to 5. Move away from the wall and walk around the room for 10 steps, trying

to maintain the correct body position. Go to the wall again, press your back against it and see if you succeeded.

Do the exerciseFive times.

2. Stand on the floor, straighten your back, put your feet shoulder-width apart. Put your hands on your belt. Without straining the neck muscles, turn your head to the right. Try to look over your right shoulder without turning your body. Turn your head to the left, again trying to look over your shoulder. Make 5 smooth turns in both directions, then 5 at a faster pace, and again 5 slow ones.

3. Stand on the floor, straighten your back, put your feet shoulder-width apart. Put your hands on your belt. Without straining the muscles of the neck, tilt your head forward. Try to touch your chest with your chin, do not raise your shoulders. Tilt your head back, stretch the back of your head to the shoulder blades. Perform 5 smooth back and forth bends, 5 at a faster pace, and again 5 slow ones.

4. Stand on the floor, straighten your back, put your feet shoulder-width apart. Extend your arms straight out in front of you. Cross and spread your arms, each time moving your arms further to the sides. Make sure your arms remain straight. Do the exercise 10-30 times.

5. Stand on the floor, straighten your back, put your feet shoulder-width apart. Bend your elbows at chest level, relax your hands and shake them for 15 seconds. Rotate your hands at the wrists - 10 times in one direction, 10 in the other.

6. Stand on the floor, straighten your back, put your feet shoulder-width apart. Lower your arms freely along the body. Take a breath. Exhaling, tilt the body to the right, moving the right hand down the surface of the thigh, and the left hand up the side of the body. Inhaling, return to the starting position. Do the exercise on the other side. Do 5-10

slopes in eachside.

7. Stand on the floor, straighten your back, put your legs wider. Lower your arms freely along the body. Take a breath. Exhaling, tilt the body

forward, trying to touch the floor with your palms. As you inhale, rise, put your hands on your belt and bend back at the waist. Perform 5-10 forward-backward bends.

8. Stand on the floor, straighten your back, put your feet shoulder-width apart. Put your hands on your belt. Rotate the body - 10-20 circles clockwise, 10-20 - against.

9. Stand on the floor, straighten your back, put your feet shoulder-width apart. Put your hands on your belt. Rotate the pelvis - 10-20 circles clockwise, 10-20 - against.

10. Stand on the floor, straighten your back, legs together, hands freely lower along the body. Raise your right leg, bending it at the knee. Try to raise your knee as high as possible. Lower your right leg and lift your left. Repeat the exercise 10-15 times for each leg.

11. Stand on the floor, straighten your back, legs together, hands freely lower along the body. Bend your right leg at the knee, touching the buttock with the heel. Lower your right leg and bend your left. Repeat the exercise 10-15 times for each leg.

12. Sit on the floor, stretch your straight legs in front of you. Keep your back straight, turn your shoulders. Place your palms on the floor just behind your buttocks. Bend your toes towards your foot. Straighten your fingers, spread them apart as wide as possible. Repeat the exercise 10 times.

13. Sit on the floor, stretch your straight legs in front of you. Keep your back straight, turn your shoulders. Bend the right leg at the knee, place the right foot on the base of the left thigh and hold the ankle with the left hand. With your right hand, gently press on your knee, trying to bring it closer to the floor. Perform 20-30 clicks. Change your leg and repeat the exercise.

Warm-up, complex2

1. Stand on the floor, straighten your back, put your feet shoulder-width apart. Put your hands on your belt. Without straining the neck muscles, rotate your head - 5 circles clockwise, 5 - counterclockwise. Repeat the exercise.

2. Stand on the floor, straighten your back, put your feet shoulder-width apart. Bend your arms at the elbows at chest level and connect the hands into the lock, turn the body to the right, stretching your arms and turning the clasped palms away from you. Return to starting position. Stretch your arms out in front of you. Return to starting position. Turn to the left, extending your arms. Return to starting position. Stretch your arms up with your head thrown back

back. Do the exercise 5-10 times.

3. Squat down. Wrap your arms around your shins and press your head to your knees. Gently lower yourself onto your buttocks and lean back. Roll back and forth for 10-15 seconds.

4. Get down on the floor on your knees, do not sit on your heels with your buttocks. Raise your straight arms up. Get down on the floor on the right, take your straight arms to the left. Raise your hands up, rise from the floor and move to the left. Take your hands to the right. Do the exercise 5-15 times.

5. Lie on the floor on your backstretch your legs, lay your arms freely along the body, tear your right leg off the floor and lift it vertically up. Count to 5, lower your leg. Repeat the exercise with the other leg. Perform the exercise 5-15 times for each leg.

6. Sit on the floor, stretch your straight legs in front of you. Keep your back straight, turn your shoulders. Place your palms on the floor just behind your buttocks. Stretch your toes forward. Pull your socks up. Repeat the exercise 10 times.

7. Sit on the floor, stretch your straight legs in front of you. Keep your back straight, turn your shoulders. Bend your knees and pull your heels towards your groin. Spread your knees to the sides. Grasp your feet with your hands and with springy movements, try to lower your knees and hips to the floor. Make 20-30 movements.

Warm-up, complex 3 (self-massage)

These exercises, performed while sitting, are recommended for debilitated children at the initial stage of yoga.

1. Place your right palm on the back of your neck and, moving your palm in a circle, make rubbing movements. Start with light stroking and move on to more intense movements, with pressure. Perform 10-15 movements with the right and left hand.
2. Put your hands on your belt and rotate your shoulder joints - 5 times forward, 5 times back. Place your right hand on your left shoulder and rub it for 15 seconds. Change hands and rub your right shoulder.
3. Lean forward a little, put your arms bent at the elbows behind your back, clench your fists and rub the surface of your back with them from the middle to the sacrum. Move your fists up and down and right to left for 20 seconds.
4. Place both palms on the knee of the bent right leg. Moving your palms in a circle, rub your knee for 20 seconds.
5. Bend your right leg at the knee and pull the foot towards you. Lay down

right foot on the left thigh and clasp it with your fingers. Stretch your right toes, foot, heel and ankle. Holding the foot with one hand, rotate it in the ankle - 10 times in one direction, 10 times in the other. Change legs.

Asanas

1. Tadasana (Samasthiti). Mountain Pose

The word "tada" in the name of the pose is translatedlike "mountain".

The word "sama" means "straight, vertical", and "sthiti" is translated as "immobility".

Thus, the name of the pose can be translated as "Direct fixed stance, mountain position."

This pose is considered the main standing asana.

herthe performance of all other vertical asanas begins.

Asana technique

1. Stand on the floor, straighten your back, connect your feet, stretch your toes. Distribute your body weight evenly over the entire foot.
2. Tighten your thigh muscles by tightening the muscles at the back of your thighs and kneecaps.
3. Draw in your stomach, straighten your shoulders, expanding your chest. Stretch your spine up as much as possible, look straight ahead.
4. Stretch out your handsalong the body.

The effect of asana on the body

Tadasana promotes the formation of correct posture and teaches you to pay attention to the position of your body.

Proper weight distribution in this position is a good prevention of flat feet.

This position of the body improves the flow of energy and metabolic processes in the body, normalizes the blood supply to the brain, therefore, improves memory, attention, and sharpens the mind.

2. Vrikshasana. Tree Pose

The word "vriksha" is translated into Russian as "tree".

Asana technique

1. Stand in Tadasana (Mountain Pose, p. 48).
2. Bend the left leg at the knee and place the left foot on the inner surface of the right thigh as close to the groin as possible with the toes down. The left knee points to the left.
3. Raise your straight arms through the sides up and connect them with your palms above your head.
4. Breathe deeply and evenly. Count to 5. Slowly return to the starting position.
5. Do the exercise with your right leg.

The effect of asana on the body

Vrikshasana is very beneficial for developing a sense of balance. This asana strengthens the muscles of the legs and helps to achieve correct posture.

Asana is very useful for developing a sense of balance.

3. Utthita trikonasana. Extended Triangle Pose

The word "utthita" is translated as "stretched". Trikonasana means triangle. The name of the asana is translated as "Elongated Triangle Pose".

Asana technique

1. Stand in Tadasana (Mountain Pose, p. 48).
2. Take a deep breath. In a jump, spread your legs at a distance of

about 1 m. Raise your arms to the sides to shoulder level (palms to the floor).

3. Turn your right foot 90 degrees to the right. Turn your left foot slightly to the right. Stretch your legs, straining your knees.
4. As you exhale, tilt the body to the right, lowering the right palm to the ankle of the right leg. Place your palm on the floor behind your right foot. If you can't reach the floor with your palm, place it on the shin of your right leg.
5. Hold your left hand up, fingers to the sky. Make sure that the back of the legs, pelvis and upper back are in the same plane.
6. Turn your head up and focus on the thumb of your left hand. Tighten the muscles of the right leg, pulling up the knee.
7. Count to 5. Breathe calmly. On an inhale, slowly return to the starting position with legs apart. Do the exercise on the other side.
8. As you exhale, jump back into Mountain Pose.(Tadasan).

The effect of asana on the body

Trikonasana is very useful for the proper development and strengthening of the muscles of the legs and the appearance of mobility of all joints of the lower extremities. This position of the body is also useful for the development of the chest.

Regular use of this asana helps to get rid of pain in the neck and back.

4. Parivritta trikonasana. Extended Triangle Pose

The word "parivritta" is translated as "turned around, back." This asana is called the Unfolded Triangle Pose and is the reverse of Utthita Trikonasana.

Asana technique

1. Stand in Tadasana (Mountain Pose, p. 48).
2. While inhaling in a jump, spread your legs to the sides by 80–90 cm. Raise your arms to the sides parallel to the floor, palms down.
3. Turn the foot of the right leg to the right side by 90 °. Turn the foot of the left leg to the right side by 60 °. Stretch your left leg and tighten your knee.

3. As you exhale, turn your body and left leg to the right, bend over and lower your left arm down. Try to place your palm on the floor behind your right foot.
4. Stretch your right arm vertically up, so that both hands are on the same line. Turn your head to the right and look at the fingers of your right hand.
5. Breathe freely. Count to 5. Slowly return to the starting position. Do the exercise on the other side.
6. Exhale and jump back into Mountain Pose.(Tadasan).

The effect of asana on the body

Performing this asana has a beneficial effect on the tone of the muscles of the legs, thighs and hamstrings. This exercise is very useful for the spine and back muscles, relieves pain and promotes the formation of correct posture.

This position of the body causes increased blood circulation in the lower spine, improving the functioning of the pelvic organs.

Expansion of the chest normalizes the work of the respiratory system.

5. Utthita parshvakonasana. Utthita parshvakonasana. Sharp Angle Pose

The word "parshva" is translated as "side", "kona" means "corner".

The name of the asana can be translated as "Pose of a sharpcorner."

Asana technique

1. Stand in Tadasana (Mountain Pose, p. 48).
2. While inhaling, jump your legs apart by 110–120 cm. Raise your arms to the sides to shoulder level (palms to the floor).
3. On a smooth exhalation, turn the right foot to the right by 90 °. Turn your left foot slightly to the right. Tighten the muscles of your left leg.
4. Bend your right leg at the knee, lowering down until your thigh is parallel to the floor. The lower leg and thigh should form a right angle.
5. Lower your right hand down and place it on the floor behind your right foot. Lower your right armpit to your right knee. Stretch your left hand obliquely up over your right ear. Look up.
6. Tighten the muscles of the lower back and tendons under the knees, bring the chest back and up. Stretch your whole body. Make sure that the legs, pelvis and chest are located in the same plane, the spine is maximally extended.
7. Breathe calmly and deeply.Count up to 5.
8. While inhaling, slowly return to the starting position with thefeet. Do the exercise on the other side.
9. Exhale and jump back into Mountain Pose.(Tadasan).

The effect of asana on the body

Utthita Parshvakonasana noticeably improves the tone of the thighs, knees and shins, helps to eliminate some defects in the development of the lower extremities, and improves the functioning of the joints.

This exercise is useful for the chest and normalization of intestinal motility. Regular practice of this asana makes the waist slim and the hips elastic.

6. Parivritta parshvakonasana. Acute angle pose with a turn

The name of this asana is translated as "Pose of an acute angle with a turn."

Asana technique

1. Stand in Tadasana (Mountain Pose, p. 48).
2. While inhaling, jump your legs apart by 100–110 cm. Raise your straight arms to the sides with your palms down to a position parallel to the floor.
3. Turn the foot of the right foot to the right side by 90°, the foot of the left foot by 60°. Stretch your left leg and tighten. Bend your right knee so that your right thigh is parallel to the floor. The shin and thigh of the right leg should form a right angle.
4. As you exhale, turn the body, transferring the left hand over the knee of the right leg. The left armpit should touch the right knee from the outside. Place the palm of your left hand on the floor outside of the foot of your right foot.
5. Rotate the body by raising the right hand forward and up over the right ear. Look at the fingers of your right hand. Brace your left knee.
6. Breathe freely. Count to 5. Slowly return to the starting position. Do the exercise on the other side.

The effect of asana on the body

This asana has a very intense effect on the whole body. A strong contraction of the abdominal organs has a beneficial effect on digestion and intestinal motility. This position of the body causes increased blood circulation in the spine.

An acute angle with a turn, becausethat the body is deployed

7. Virabhadrasana I. Warrior Pose I

This asana got its name from the name of a mighty warrior whom the god Shiva created from his hair. Often its name is translated as -

"Warrior Pose".

Asana technique

1. Stand in Tadasana (Mountain Pose, p. 48).
2. Through the sides, raise your straight arms up and connect them with your palms above your head.
3. Inhale, jumpspread your legs to the sides by 110–120 cm.
4. Exhale as you turn your bodyto the left, turn the left foot to the left side by 90 °, turn the right foot slightly to the left.
5. Gently bend your left knee until your left thigh is parallel to the floor. In this case, the left thigh and left lower leg should form a right angle. Make sure that the knee does not protrude too far forward.
6. Stretch your left leg, tighten your knee.
7. The body and face are turned to the right. Tilt your head back, arching your back. Pull the joined hands up. Look up at your palms.

8. Breathe evenly and calmly. Count to 5. Slowly return to the
starting position with legs apart. Do the exercise on the other
side. Exhale and return to PoseMountains (Tadasanu).

People with cardiovascular disorders should practice this pose with great
care and do not stay in it for more than 5-10 seconds.

The effect of asana on the body

The expansion of the chest in this asana normalizes the functioning of the
respiratory system.

This posture is very beneficial for developing the mobility of the neck,
shoulders and back, and it has a tonic effect on the knees and lower legs.

Regular practice of this asana helps to get rid of excess fat deposits in the
pelvic region.

8. Virabhadrasana II. Warrior Pose II

Asana technique

1. Stand in Tadasana (Mountain Pose, p. 48).
2. Inhaling, jump spread your legs to the sides by 110-120 cm.
Raise your arms to the sides parallel to the floor, palms
down.
3. Turn the body to the right, turn the right foot 90 ° to the
right side, slightly turn the left foot to the right. Stretch
your left leg and tighten the muscles under your knee.
4. As you exhale, bend your right knee so that your right
thigh is parallel to the floor. In this case, the right thigh

and right shin should form a right angle. Do not push your right knee forward.

5. Stretch your arms out to the sides.
6. Turn your head to the right, look at the right hand. Make sure that the pelvis, shoulders and back of the legs are in the same plane.
7. Breathe evenly and calmly. Count to 5. While inhaling, slowly return to the starting position with legs apart. Do the exercise on the other side.
8. Exhale and return to PoseMountains (Tadasanu).

The effect of asana on the body

Regular practice of this asana makes the legs strong. andbeautiful, their joints are flexible and mobile.

This pose is useful for maintaining the tone of the abdominal muscles.

Posture makes legs strongand beautiful

9. Virabhadrasana III. Warrior Pose III

This asana is a continuation of Virabhadrasana, but involves a greater load on the muscles.

Asana technique

1. Stand in Tadasana (Mountain Pose, p. 48).
2. Perform Virabhadrasana I (Warrior Pose) to the right.
3. As you exhale, tilt your body forward and lie with your chest on the thigh of your right leg, stretch your arms forward with joined palms.

Take two deep breaths in and out.

4. As you exhale, swing forward a little and lift your left leg off the floor. Straighten your right leg and tighten your muscles. Raise your left leg to a position parallel to the floor. The left leg, body and outstretched arms should be in one line.

5. Breathe freely. Count to 5. Slowly return toVirabhadrasana I (Warrior Pose). Do the exercise on the other side.

The effect of asana on the body

Practicing this asana is a great way to develop a sense of balance and harmony, improve your posture and lighten your gait. The muscles of the abdominal cavity in this position are constantly in good shape, the legs become strong and beautiful.

10. Ardha Chandrasana. Crescent Pose

Asana technique

1. Stand in Tadasana (Mountain Pose, p. 48) and assume the position of Utthita Trikonasana (Elongated Triangle Pose, p. 52) to the right.

2. As you exhale, place the palm of your right hand on the floor at a distance of 20–

25 cm from the right leg, bend the right leg at the knee, move the left foot to the right.

3. Take two breaths in and out. As you exhale, lift your left leg off the floor and lift it up. Extend your right leg and arm, resting them on the floor. Most of the weight of the body should be on the leg, the arm serves to maintain balance.

4. Place the palm of your left hand on the thigh of your left leg. Extend your left leg. Straighten your shoulders, turning your chest slightly to the left.
5. Breathe freely. Count to 5. Slowly return to the starting position. Do the exercise on the other side.

The effect of asana on the body

This asana is very useful for strengthening the muscles of the legs and lower back. Performing this exercise has a beneficial effect on the condition of the stomach.

11. Utthita hasta padangushthasana. Outstretched Hand and Big Toe

The name of this asana is formed by the words "utthita" -

"stretched", "hasta", which means "hand", and "padangustha", which translates as "big toe".

Asana technique

1. Stand in Tadasana (Mountain Pose, p. 48).
2. As you exhale, bend your right leg at the knee, lift it up. Grasp the big toe of the right foot with the fingers of the right hand.
3. Place your left hand on your waistband. Take two deep breaths in and out.
4. As you exhale, raise your right arm and stretch your left leg up. Take two deep breaths in and out.
5. Grab your right foot or lower leg with both hands and lift your

leg as high as you can. Do not bend your right leg at the knee. Take two deep breaths in and out.

6.   Try to pull your leg to your head and press your face to your knee. Count to 5. Slowly return to the starting position. Do the exercise with the other leg.

The effect of asana on the body

This asana is very effective for stretching the leg muscles and developing a sense of balance.

12.

Parshvottanasana. Intense Lateral Stretch Pose

Asana technique

1.   Stand in Tadasana (Mountain Pose, p. 48). Take a deep breath and move your body slightly forward.

2 Bend your elbows, bring them behind your back and, as you exhale, join your palms in the Indian gesture of greeting and respect "namaste". Pull your shoulders back. Make sure that the palms are located between the shoulder blades.

3.   Take a deep breath and jump your legs apart by 80-100 cm. Exhale smoothly.

4. As you inhale, turn your body to the right. Rotate the right foot to the right side by 90°. Make sure that the toes and heel of the right foot are in line with the body. Turn the foot of the left leg to the right by 75°. Stretch your left leg and tighten your knee. Tilt your head back.
5. As you exhale, lean forward, trying to touch your right knee with your head. Stretch your back and neck as much as possible.
6. Breathe evenlyand calmly. Count up to 5.
7. While inhaling, moving the body around the pelvis, smoothly move it to the left knee, turning the left foot 90° to the left side, the right one - 75°. Straighten up, tilt your head back, arching your back.
8. As you exhale, tilt your body forward, trying to touch your left knee with your head. Breathe freely. Count up to 5.
9. Move the body and head to the center, place the feet parallel to each other. Raise the body.
10. Exhale and jump to connect your legs. Lowerarms.

If it is difficult for you to put your palms together in "namaste", join your hands behind your back, clasping your wrist with the other with one hand or clasping your left elbow with your right palm and your right elbow with your left.

The effect of asana on the body

Practicing this asana is very beneficial for developing mobility

joints of the legs and pelvis, giving flexibility to the spine and wrists, developing the correct posture. In an inclined position, the work of the abdominal organs is normalized. Pulling the shoulders back improves the functioning of the respiratory system.

Lateral traction

13. Prasarita Padottanasana I. Wide Feet Pose I

The word "prasarita" is translated as "stretched",

"straightened", "pada" means "foot". The name of this asana can be translated as "Pose with feet wide apart".

Asana technique

1. Stand in Tadasana (Mountain Pose, p. 48).
2. Take a deep breath and place your palms on your belt. Spread your legs as wide as possible. Make sure your feet are parallel.
3. Tighten your leg muscles, pull your kneecaps up. As you exhale, lean forward and place your palms on the floor. The arms should be perpendicular to the floor.
4. While inhaling, raise your head, slightly arching your back in the lower back. Look ahead.
5. Take a deep breath. Bend your elbows and lower your head on the floor between your palms. Do not lean on your head - the weight of the body remains on the legs.
6. Breathe freely. Count to 5. Slowly return to the starting position.
7. Exhale and jump back into Mountain Pose.(Tadasan).

The effect of asana on the body

Performing this exercise contributes to a good stretching of the hamstrings, helps to get rid of the feeling of fatigue and improve the functioning of the digestive organs.

14. Prasarita padottanasana II. Wide Feet Pose II

This asana is an advanced version of Prasarita Padottanasana.

I.

Asana technique

1. Stand in Tadasana (Mountain Pose, p. 48).
2. Take a deep breath and place your palms on your belt. Spread your legs

as wide as possible. Make sure thatfeet were parallel.

3. Tighten your leg muscles, tighten your kneecaps up. Bend your elbows, bring them behind your back and join your palms in

"namaste".

5. Take a deep breath. Lean forward and place your head on the floor between your palms. Do not lean on your head - the weight of the body remains on the legs.
6. Breathe freely. Count to 5. Slowly return to the starting position.
7. Exhale and jump back into Mountain Pose.(Tadasan).

The effect of asana on the body

This position of the body not only tightens the muscles and tendons of the legs, but also significantly increases blood flow to the torso and head. This asana has a beneficial effect on the work of the gastrointestinal tract, in particular, improving digestion.

15. Parighasana. Bolt Pose

The word "parigha" is translated as "bolt" or "beam".

Asana technique

1. Get on the floor on your knees, bring your legs together.
2. Straighten your right leg to the side, toes to the right. Don't bend your knee.
3. As you inhale, raise your straight arms to the sides with your palms down. Take two breaths in and out.
4. As you exhale, tilt your body and lower your hand to the right, towards the outstretched leg. Try to place the forearm of the right hand on the shin of the right leg, the hand of the right hand on the right ankle. Raise your left hand up.
5. Tilt your head until your eardoes not touch the right shoulder. Reach with your left hand to your right, so that the left ear touches the left shoulder.
6. Breathe freely. Count to 5. Slowly return to the starting position. Do the exercise on the other side.

The effect of asana on the body

Practicing this asana is very beneficial for stretching the pelvic region and spine. Stretching the peritoneum on one side with simultaneous compression on the other provides an internal massage of the abdominal organs.

16. Ushtrasana. camel pose

The name of this asana is derived from the word "ushtra"- "camel".

Asana technique

1. Get on the floor on your knees; connect the feet, knees and hips. Don't put your buttocks on your heels.
2. Place your palms on your hips at the back, stretch your hips (thighs and shins should form a right angle) and arch your back back.
3. Put your hands on your heels, trying to cover with your palmsfeet.
4. Lean on your hands, tilt your head back and arch your back. Tighten the muscles of the buttocks, bringing the pelvis forward.
5. Breathe freely. Count to 10. Slowly return to the starting position.

The effect of asana on the body

Regular practice of this asana will ensure good posture and relieve back pain.

17. Utkatasana. Power Pose

Asana technique

1. Stand in Tadasana (Mountain Pose, p. 48). Raise your straight arms up and join your palms above your head.
2. As you exhale, slowly bend your knees as you lower yourself down. Stop when your thighs are parallel to the floor.
3. Do not tilt your body forward, try to tilt your chest back.
4. Breathe freely. Count to 5. Return slowly

The effect of asana on the body

This asana is very useful for developing the muscles of the legs and correcting small defects in their structure. The upward movement of the diaphragm in this posture is helpful in normalizing the functioning of the heart muscle and abdominal organs.

Regular performance of this exercise significantly increases the mobility of the shoulder joints.

18. Padangushthasana. Standing pose with the grip of the big toes

The name of this asana is formed by combining two words: "pada", meaning "foot", and "angushtha", which means big toe.

Asana technique

1. Stand in Tadasana (Mountain Pose, p. 48). Place your feet at a distance of 20-30 cm from each other.
2. As you exhale, gently lean forward. Lower your palms to the floor and clasp your big toes with your middle, index, and thumbs.
3. Bend your back in the lower back, raise your head, pull the diaphragm up. Stretch your shoulder blades and do not bend your knees. Take two breaths in and out.
4. As you exhale, lower your head to your knees. Tighten your knees, pull your big toes up with your hands, but do not tear them off the floor.
5. Breathe freely. Count to 5. Slowly return to the starting position.

The effect of asana on the body

This position of the body has a tonic effect on the abdominal organs - the secretion of digestive juices increases, the work of the spleen and liver is activated, intestinal motility improves, flatulence disappears.

19. Padahastasana. Back of Legs Maximum Stretch Pose

Asana technique

1. Stand in Tadasana (Mountain Pose, p. 48). Place your feet at a distance of 20-30 cm from each other.
2. As you exhale, tilt your body forward, place your hands on the floor, leading under the feet from the outside. Soles and palms should touch.
3. Raise your head and arch your backdon't bend your knees.

The effect of asana on the body

In this asana, the rectum and bladder are actively affected. Also, this exercise is useful for improving the functioning of the liver, spleen and kidneys.

Regular performance of this exercise significantly increases the flexibility of the spine.

20. Uttanasana. Intense Spine Stretch Pose

The particle "ut" is used to denote deliberate intensity, the word "tan" is translated as "stretching". In this position, there is a deliberate increased stretching of the spine.

Asana technique

1. Stand in Tadasana (Mountain Pose, p. 48).
2. As you exhale, tilt your body forward, lowering your fingers to the floor. Place your palms on the floor behind your heels. Make sure that your legs do not bend at the knees.
3. Raise your head up. Make twoinhale and exhale.
4. As you exhale, lower your head, trying to touch your knees with your face. Pull your kneecaps up.
5. Breathe freely. Count to 5. Slowly return to the starting position.

The effect of asana on the body

Performing this asana is beneficial for the normal functioning of the liver, kidneys, spleen, for relieving pain in the abdomen and for the menstruation period in women.

Even breathing in this position helps to cope with an increase in heart rate, stretching the spine stimulates the nerves of the back.

Prolonged stay in this position has a positive effect on brain function, eliminates depressive states.

21. Urdhva prasarita ekapadasana. Bent over with Leg Raised Up

The name of the asana consists of the words "urdhva", which translates as

"upper, high, vertical", "prasarita" - "stretched out", "eka", which means "one", and "pada" - "foot".

Asana technique

1. Stand in Tadasana (Mountain Pose, p. 48).
2. As you exhale, tilt your body forward, trying to touch your knees with your head. Place your palms on the floor next to your feet.
3. Raise your left leg back to the maximum height, try to keep the extended toe of the raised leg looking up. Tighten the muscles in both legs.
4. Breathe freely. Count to 5. While inhaling, lower your leg to the floor and slowly straighten up. Do the exercise with the other leg.

The effect of asana on the body

This pose helps to strengthen the muscles of the legs and makes the pelvic area more "tight".

22. Ardha baddha padmottanasana. Half Lotus Pose Standing On One Leg

The name of this asana is formed by a combination of the words "ardha", which means "half", "baddha", which translates as "bound, held", "padma" - "lotus" and "uttana" - "intense stretching".

Asana technique

1. Stand in Tadasana (Mountain Pose, p. 48).
2. As you inhale, bend your left leg at the knee and lift your foot up. Place your left foot on your right thigh.
3. Holding the left foot with the right hand, bring the left hand behind the back, bring the brush out from the opposite side and grab the big toe of the left foot with the fingers.
4. As you exhale, lean forward. Place the palm of your right hand on the floor in front of your right foot. Raise your head and try to arch your back. If you find it difficult to hold your left leg, release your left hand and lower it to the floor next to your right.
5. Try to bend as low as possible - stretch your head to the knee of your right leg.
6. Breathe freely. Count to 5. Slowly return to the starting position. Do the exercise with the other leg.

The effect of asana on the body

This pose is very beneficial for developing the flexibility and mobility of the knee joints. The contraction of the abdominal organs in this position normalizes intestinal motility.

23. Garudasana. Eagle Pose

The word "garuda" is translated as "eagle". Also in Indian mythology, this is the name of the lord of birds, who wears the god Vishnu on his back.

Asana technique

1. Stand in Tadasana.
2. A littlebend your right leg at the knee.
3. Cross your legs withleft thigh to right. Move the left leg around the right, pressing the shin of the left leg against the shin of the right. Pass the toe of the left foot behind the right shin and hook on it.

7. 1. Bend your elbows at chest level. Place your right elbow on the inner surface of your left hand near the cubital fossa. Move the right palm slightly to the right, the left to the left and connect them.
2. Breathe freely. Count to 5. Slowly return to the starting position. Do the exercise on the other side.

The effect of asana on the body

This exercise is very useful for developing the mobility of the shoulder joints and strengthening the ankles.

Garuda in Indian mythology is the name of the lord of birds, who wears the god Vishnu on his back.

24. Vatayanasana. horse pose

The name of this asana is translated as "Horse Pose".

Asana technique

1. Sit on the floor, stretch your straight legs in front of you. Bend your left leg at the knee, pull the foot towards you. Place your left foot on your right thigh, placing your heel as close to your stomach as possible.
2. Rest your palms on the floor on the sides of your buttocks. As you exhale, lift your pelvis off the floor, lower your left knee to the floor. Bend your right leg at the knee at a right angle, put your foot on the floor.
3. Straighten your back and raise your arms. Maintain balance by moving the pelvis slightly forward, but do not tilt the body.
4. Bend your elbows at chest level. Place your right hand with your shoulder (near the elbow) on the antecubital fossa of your left hand. Circle the right hand around the left and join the palms.
5. Breathe freely. Count to 5. Slowly return to the starting position. Do the exercise on the other side. Lie on the floor on your back and relax.

The effect of asana on the body

This asana is very beneficial for developing mobility in the pelvis and sacrum.

25. Shalabhasana. Locust Pose

The word "shalabha" is translated as "locust".

Asana technique

1. Lie on the floor on your stomach, stretch. Stretch your arms back, lower your face down.

2. As you exhale, lift your legs, arms, head, shoulders and chest off the floor and lift to the maximum height. Make sure your legs are straight and tight. The weight of the body should remain on the stomach. Tighten the muscles in your thighs and buttocks.

3. Pull your arms back,tense back muscles.

4. Breathe freely. Count to 5. Slowly return to the starting position.

The effect of asana on the body

Regular practice of this asana helps to get rid of fromflatulence, elimination of disorders of the digestive system.

This exercise increases the flexibility of the spine, relieves back pain.

26. Crocodile pose. Makarasana

floor. *This asana is a variant of Shalabhasana (Locust Pose).*

Asana technique

1. Lie on the floor on your stomach, stretch your arms along the body, lower your face to

2. Place your hands on the back of your head with your palms. Get

straight off the floor

clenched legs, head, shoulders and chest and liftto the maximum height.

3. Breathe freely. Count to 5. Slowly return to the starting position.

The effect of asana on the body

Performing this exercise has the same effect as Locust Pose
(Shalabhasana).

27. Dhanurasana. bow pose

*The name of the asana is derived from the word "dhanu" - "bow", since the
position of the body in this pose resembles a bow with a stretched bowstring.*

Asana technique

1. Lie on the floor on your stomach, place your hands along the body
    with palms down, lower your face to the floor.
2. As you exhale, bend both legs at the knees. Raise your arms and
    clasp your ankles with your palms. Take two breaths in and out.
3. As you exhale with your hands, pull your legs up and towards your
    head, tearing your chest off the floor and arching your back.
4. Tilt your head back. Do not touch the floor with the pelvis and ribs,
    the weight of the body should fall on the stomach.
5. Count to 5. As you exhale, slowly return to starting position.

The effect of asana on the body

Regular practice of this asana makes the spine mobile and flexible, and also has a tonic effect on the abdominal organs.

28. Parshva dhanurasana. Side bow pose

This asana is Bow Pose done on the side.

Asana technique

1. Lie on the floor on your stomach. Perform Dhanurasana (Bow Pose, p. 98). Take a deep breath.
2. As you exhale, gently roll over to your left side. Arch your back by stretching your legs. Count to 5. Return to regular Dhanurasana. Roll over to the right side. Count to 5. While lying on your side, hold your ankles firmly.
3. Return to starting position. Relax.

The effect of asana on the body

Rolling from side to side in this asana, you gently massage the abdominal organs.

This exercise is also very useful for developing the flexibility of the spine and joints, forming the correct posture and strengthening the legs.

29. Chaturanga dandasana. Staff Pose

spine flexibility

The name of this asana is formed by the words "chatur", which means

"four", "anga" - "part", "limb", and "danda", which translates as "staff".

Asana technique

1. Lie on the floor on your stomach, bend your arms at the elbows, place your palms on the floor at chest level, stretch your legs and strain.
2. Spread your legs 20-30 cm apart.
3. As you exhale, lift your entire body off the floor. Leaning on the palms and toes, try to keep the body in a position parallel to the floor.
4. Breathe freely. Count to 5. Slowly lower yourself to the floor. Stretch your arms along the body. Relax.

The effect of asana on the body

This asana is useful for developing the wrists, strengthening the muscles of the arms and the abs.

30. Cobra Pose. Bhujangasana

The name of the pose is derived from the word "bhujanga", which translates as "snake".

Asana technique

1. Lie on your stomach, lower your face to the floor. Connect

the feet of the outstretched legs, pull the socks, tighten the
knees.
2. Bend your elbows, place your palms on the floor at chest
level.
3. As you exhale, leaning on your palms, tear your head,
shoulders and chest off the floor and raise your body. Take
two breaths in and out.
4. On inspiration, the back will rot, tearing the stomach off
the floor. Tilt your head back, tighten your hips and
buttocks.
5. Breathe freely. Count to 5. As you exhale, gently bend your
elbows and return to the starting position.

The effect of asana on the body

This asana is very useful for toning the spine area and increasing its
flexibility.

31. Adho muksha (mukha) svanasana. Downward Facing Dog Pose

The combination of the words "adho mukha" is translated as "face down", and

shvana means dog.

Asana technique

1. Lie on the floor on your stomach, spread your straight
legs to the sides by 20–30 cm.
2. Bend your arms at the elbows and place your palms on

the floor at chest level with your fingers forward.
3. As you exhale, lift your pelvis off the floor and lift it up. Straightening your arms, tear your legs, stomach, chest off the floor. Move your head towards your feet and lower your crown to the floor. Bend your arms at the shoulder joints, stretch your back.
4. Do not bend your knees, do not take your feet off the floor.
5. Breathe freely. Count to 5. While inhaling, raise your head, stretch forward and slowly lower yourself to the floor. Stretch your arms along your body and relax.

The effect of asana on the body

This posture helps to quickly get rid of physical and mental fatigue, causes a powerful surge of energy.

Regular practice of this asana strengthens the muscles of the legs and improves their shape. Useful exercise for the spine and shoulder joints.

32. Paripurna navasana. Boat pose

The word "paripurna" means "whole, complete, complete",

"nava" is translated as "vessel, boat". The name of this asana means

"Fullboat pose.

Asana technique

1. Sit on the floor, straighten your legs. Place your

palms on the floor near your buttocks, fingers forward. Roll your shoulders, straighten your back.

2. Take a deep breath and exhale. Lift your legs off the floor, moving your body back a little. Bending your knees, raise your legs to a 60° angle. The feet should be above the head. Do not lean on the floor with your lower back - only the buttocks should touch the floor.

3. Stretch your straight arms forward, parallel to the floor, palms facing each other.

4. Breathe freely. Count to 5. Slowly return to the starting position. Relax.

The effect of asana on the body

This asana strengthens the muscles of the legs, back and abs, and also reduces fat deposits in the abdomen and waist. This exercise is useful for normalizing the work of the intestines and kidneys, getting rid of flatulence.

33. Ardha navasana. Half boat pose

The word ardha means half.The name of the asana is translated as

"Half Boat Pose".

Asana technique

1. Sit on the floor, stretch your straight legs forward. join your hands in a lock at the back of your head.

2. Take a deep breath and exhale. Lift your legs off

the floor, moving your body back a little. Bending your knees, raise your legs at an angle of 30–40°. Feet should be at head level. Do not lean on the floor with your lower back - only the buttocks should touch the floor. Feel the tension in your abdominal and lower back muscles.

4. Breathe freely. Count to 5. Slowly return to the starting position. Relax.

The effect of asana on the body

This exercise is very useful for the normalization of the liver, spleen and gallbladder. The tension of the muscles of the legs, abs and back during the performance of this asana increases their endurance.

34. Gomukasana (gomukhasana). Cow head pose

The name of this asana is usually translated as "Cow Head Pose", since the word "go" means "cow" and "mukha" means "face".

Asana technique

1. Sit on the floorstretch straight legs in front of you.
2. Place your palms on the floor and lift your buttocks off the floor.
3. Bend your left leg under you and lower your buttocks onto your foot. Bend your right leg at the knee and place your thigh on top of your left. Raise your buttocks and, helping yourself with your hands, try to connect your shins and feet.
4. Raise your right arm and bend at the elbow above your head. Bend your left arm at the elbow and bring it behind your back from below.

Join your palms behind your back at the level of your shoulder
blades.
5.   Breathe freely. Count to 5. Slowly return to the starting position. Do
the exercise on the other side.

The effect of asana on the body

This exercise is useful for developing the elasticity of the joints of the legs
and arms, strengthening the muscles of the legs and opening the chest.

35. Siddhasana. Perfect Pose (Sage Pose)

The word "siddha" is translated as "prophet", "sage".

Asana technique

1.   Sit on the floorStretch straight legs in front of you.
2.   Bend your right leg at the knee. Grab the right foot with your
palms and move the heel as close to the groin as possible. Press
the foot of the right foot to the left thigh.
3.   Bend your left leg at the knee and pull your foot towards you.
Place the foot of the left leg on the shin of the right leg, placing
the heel against the pubis. Place the foot of the left leg between
the thigh and lower leg of the right.
4.   Straighten your arms. Place your palms on your knees with the
backs. Connect the thumb and index finger on each hand into a
ring. Straighten your back, look ahead.
5.   Breathe freely. Count to 5. Slowly return to the starting position.
Perform the asana by changing legs.

The effect of asana on the body

This asana is considered one of the best yoga postures for relaxation.

Regular performance of this exercise develops the mobility of the leg joints, tones the abdominal organs and has a beneficial effect on the spine.

36. Virasana. Hero Pose

The name of this pose is derived from the word "vira" - "hero",

"winner".

Asana technique

1. Sit on the floor on your knees. Spread your feet to the sides by 20-40 cm.
2. Lower your buttocks to the floor or to your feet.
3. Place your hands on your knees with the backs of your hands. Connect your thumb and index finger into a ring. Straighten your back, look ahead.
4. Breathe freely. Count to 5. Relax.

The effect of asana on the body

Performing this exercise helps to get rid of flat feet and strengthens the knees.

37. Supta Virasana. diamond pose

The word "supta" is translated as "lying". This is a variant of the Winner's Pose.

Asana technique

1. Sit on the floor on your knees. Spread your feet to the sides by 20-40 cm.
2. Lower your buttocks to the floor or to your feet.
3. On the exhale, tilt the body back and lean on the elbows andforearms on the floor.
4. Gently stretch your arms forward, dropping to the top of your head thrown back.
5. Lower your shoulders and back to the floor.
6. Stretch your arms behind your head. Don't liftshoulder blades.
7. If the pose is given to youeasy, bring your knees together.
8. Breathe deeply. Count to 5. Slowly return to the starting position. Relax.

The effect of asana on the body

This asana is very useful for stretching the pelvis and affecting the abdominal organs. Regular performance of this asana strengthens the legs and relieves fatigue after prolonged physical exertion.

afterprolonged physical activity

38. Bhekasana. Frog Pose

The word "bheka" in translation means "frog", so the name of this asana is "Frog Pose".

Asana technique

1. Lie on the floor on your stomach, put your hands along the body.
2. As you exhale, bend your knees, bringing your heels closer to your buttocks. Wrap your arms around your feet and pull your legs towards your body. Take two breaths in and out.
3. As you exhale, tear offoff the floor head, look up.
4. Place your palms on your feet with your fingers forward. Pressing with your hands, try to bring your heels closer to the floor. Forearms should be perpendicular to the floor.
5. Breathe freely. Count to 5. Slowly return to the starting position. Relax.

The effect of asana on the body

This pose strengthens the knees and relievesflat feet.

Regular performance of this exercise provides a gentle internal massage of the abdominal organs.

39. Baddha konasana. butterfly pose

The word "baddha" means "captured", and "kona" is translated as

"corner". This asana is often referred to as Shoemaker's Pose.

Asana technique

1. Sit on the floorstretch straight legs in front of you.
2. Bend your legsin my knees. Move your heels towards your groin.
3. Press your feet together with your hands. Try to keep your knees and hips on the floor.
4. Hold your feet firmly with your fingers interlocked. Straighten your shoulders, stretch your back, look straight ahead. Count up to 5.
5. Place your elbows on your knees, then press them to the floor.
6. As you exhale, tilt your body forward. Try to touch the floor with your forehead, nose, and chin.
7. Breathe freely. Count to 5. Slowly return to the starting position. Relax.

The effect of asana on the body

This asana is very useful for normalizing the functioning of the urinary and reproductive organs, as in this pose it improves blood flow in the pelvic organs.

40. Padmasana. Lotus position

This asana is well knownlike the lotus position.

Asana technique

1. Sit on the floorstretch straight legs in front of you.
2. Bend your right leg at the knee, grab your foot with your hands and pull it towards you. Place the foot of the right foot on the top of the thigh of the left foot, trying to place the heel as close to the navel as possible.
3. Bend your left kneeleg, grasp the foot with your hands and pull it towards you. Place the foot of your left foot on top of your right thigh. Pull your heel towards your navel. The feet of both legs look up.
4. Place your hands on your knees or fold your palms at chest level ("namaste").
5. Breathe freely. Count to 5. Slowly return to the starting position. Perform the exercise by changing legs.

The effect of asana on the body

Once mastered, this asana becomes one of the best postures for relaxation and relaxation.

This exercise is very useful for developing the mobility of the joints of the legs and normalizing blood circulation in the pelvic area.

41. Shanmukhi mudra. Sealing pose

"Shanmukha" (from "shan" - "six", "mukha" - "mouth") is the name of the god of war, who has six heads. The word "mudra" means "closing",

"sealing". This asana can also be called Parangmukhi Mudra, Yoni Mudra or Shambhavi Mudra.

Asana technique

1. Sit on the floor, stretch your straight legs in front of you. Take Padmasana (Lotus Pose).
2. Straighten your back, lift your chin.
3. Raise your arms bent at the elbows and bring your palms to your face. Plug your ears with your thumbs.
4. Close your eyes, but look up under your eyelids. Place the two upper phalanges of the middle and index fingers on closed eyelids. Don't force your eyes. Pull your eyelids down slightly with your middle fingers. With your index fingers, press upward on the area under the eyebrows.
5. Put the tips of your index fingers on the nostrils and press a little, narrowing the nasal passages.
6. Put the little fingers on the toplip.
7. Breathe calmly and slowly. Count to 10. Slowly lower your arms and open your eyes.

The effect of asana on the body

This asana is a wonderful posture for gaininginner peace.

42. Simhasana I. Lion Pose I

This asana - "Lion's Pose" - is dedicated to the man-lion Narasimha, in whom, according to legend, the god Vishnu was embodied.

Asana technique

1. Sit on the floor, stretch your straight legs in front of you.

2. Bend your knees and pull under you, crossing at the ankles. Lowering the buttocks on the feet - right on the left foot, left on the right foot.

3. Straighten your back and lean forward a little, transferring your body weight to your knees and hips.

4. Place your palms on your knees and lean on them. Spread your fingers apart.

5. Open your mouth as wide as possible, stick out your tongue, trying to reach your chin.

6. Open your eyes wide, look at the tip of the nose.

7. Breathe freely. Count to 10. Return to starting position. Repeat the exercise by changing legs.

The effect of asana on the body

This asana is very useful for the treatment of colds, especially sore throats. With regular exercise, halitosis disappears and the process of curing stuttering is accelerated.

43. Matsyasana. Fish Pose

This asana - "Pose of the Fish" - is dedicated to the fish, in which the god Vishnu was embodied.

Asana technique

1. Sit on the floor, stretch your straight legs in front of you. Take Padmasana (Lotus Pose).

2. Gently lower yourself onto your back. Don't take your feet off the floor.

3. Exhale as you arch your back, lifting your neck and shoulder blades off the floor. Lean on the back of your head with your head thrown back. Hold your legs with your hands.

4. Bend your elbows and lay next to your head.

5. Breathe freely. Count to 5. Slowly rise and return to the starting position. Relax.

The effect of asana on the body

This asana is extremely useful for expanding the chest and normalizing breathing. Stretching in this exercise has a beneficial effect on the condition of the thyroid gland.

This pose increases the flexibility of the spine and hip joints.

44. Baddha padmasana. Closed Lotus Pose

The word "baddha" means "grasped" - in this asana the whole body is caught by intertwined arms and legs.

Asana technique

1. Sit on the floor, stretch your straight legs in front of you. Take Padmasana (Lotus Pose). Take a deep breath.

2. As you exhale, bring your left hand behind your back and bring the brush out from the opposite side. Grasp the big toe of the left foot with the fingers of the left hand. Take a deep breath.

3. As you exhale, bring your right hand behind your back, bring your hand out on the left side and grab the big toe of your right foot with the fingers of your right hand.

4. Pull your shoulders back, bringing your shoulder blades together - this will make it easier for you to complete the exercise. First of all, grab the big toe of the foot that lies on top.

5. Stretch your neck, tilting your head back. Look up. Take 3 deep breaths and exhale. Slowly return to the starting position.

The effect of asana on the body

With a strong institution of hands behind the back, the chest expands, which has a beneficial effect on the functioning of the respiratory system.

This asana is useful for developing the flexibility of the joints and spine, correcting posture defects.

45. Supta vajrasana. Sleeping Lightning Pose

The name of this asana consists of two words "supta" - "lying" and

"Vajra", which translates as "thunderbolt".

This is a rather difficult asana that will require a lot of practice.

Asana technique

1. Sit on the floor, stretch your straight legs in front of you. Take Padmasana (Lotus Pose). Perform Baddha Padmasana. Take a deep breath.

2. As you exhale, lift your knees and hips off the floor and tilt your body back, sinking to the floor. Take 2 deep breaths and exhale.

3. Stretch your neck, arch your back, bringing your chest up, and rest your crown on the floor.

4. As you exhale, bring your knees and hips to the floor. In this asana, you touch the floor with your buttocks, arms, elbows, and crown.

5. Count to 5. Release your toes and rise. Return tostarting position. Relax. Perform the exercise by changing legs.

The effect of asana on the body

When performing this exercise, there is a strong stretching of the spine and expansion of the chest. When the neck is retracted, the normalization of the thyroid gland occurs. This asana is very useful for developing the flexibility of the hip joints.

46. Maha Mudra. great seal

The name of this asana consists of the words "maha", which translates as "great", and "mudra" - "sealing", "closing".

Asana technique

1. Sit on the floor, stretch your straight legs in front of you.

2. Bend the left leg at the knee, place the outer side of the thigh and lower leg on the floor and take it to the side. Pull the heel of the left foot as close to you as possible and place the foot on the inner surface of the right thigh. The bent and straight legs should form a right angle.

3. Stretch your hands to the toe of your right foot and grab your big toe with your fingers.

4. Tilt your body forward without lowering your chest to your leg. As you inhale, draw in your stomach and tighten your abdominal muscles. Count to 5. Exhale as you relax your muscles. Inhale, tighten your abs and pull in your stomach. Count to 5. As you exhale, relax your muscles and slowly return to the starting position. Do the exercise on the other side.

The effect of asana on the body

This exercise is very useful for normalizing the work of all organs.abdomen, kidneys and adrenal glands. This asana has a beneficial effect on women's health, ensuring the correct position of the uterus.

47. Janu shirshasana. head on knee

The name of this asana is made up of two words: "janu", which translates as "knee", and "shirsha" - head.

Asana technique

1. Sit on the floor, stretch your straight legs in front of you.

2. Bend the left leg at the knee, place the outer side of the thigh and lower leg on the floor and take it to the side. Pull the heel of the left foot as close to you as possible and place the foot on the inner surface of the right thigh.

The bent and straight legs should form an obtuse angle.

3. Stretch your arms to the toe of your right leg and grab the foot with your palms or, having put your hands behind the foot, clasp the wrist with one hand with the other. Keep your right knee off the floor.

4. As you exhale, bend your elbows and push them apart. At the same time, tilt the body and lower the head to the knee of the right leg. Extend your back and lower your chest to your right thigh.

5. Count to 5. Lower your head to the floor, first on one side, then on the other side of the knee. Make sure that the right foot does not move to the right.

6. Slowly return to the starting position. Do the exercise on the other side.

The effect of asana on the body

Performing this exercise has a beneficial effect on digestion, on the work of the spleen, liver and kidneys.

48. Parivritta Janu Sirshasana. Twisted Head To Knee Pose

The word "parivritta" is translated as "turned". Parivrtta Janu Sirshasana is the Twisted Head to Knee Pose, a variant of Janu Sirshasana.

Asana technique

1. Sit on the floor, stretch your straight legs in front of you.

2. Bend the left leg at the knee, place the outer side of the thigh and lower leg on the floor and take it to the side. Pull the heel of the left foot as close to you as possible and place the foot on the inner surface of the right thigh. The bent and straight legs should form an obtuse angle. Take two deep breaths in and out.

3. As you exhale, turning the body to the left, bend over to the right leg, bringing the right shoulder and hand in front of the knee.

4. Grasp the foot of the right foot with your right hand, stretch your left hand over the left ear and grab the foot of the right foot from the outside with your palm. Look ahead and up.

5. Try to retract the right shoulder blade and twist at the waist, lifting the left side of the back.

6. Breathe freely. Count to 5. Slowly return to the starting position. Do the exercise on the other side.

The effect of asana on the body

This asana perfectly stretches the spine, relieving pain and fatigue in the back, increasing flexibility, and improving posture.

49. Ardha baddha padma pashchimottanasana. Pose of intense stretching of the entire back of the body

The word "ardha" is translated as "half", "baddha" means

"caught", "padma" - lotus. Pashchimottanasana - A pose of intense stretching of the entire back of the body.

Asana technique

1. Sit on the floor, stretch your straight legs in front of you.

2. Bend your left leg at the knee, pull the foot towards you and place it on your right thigh with your hands. Press the left heel to the navel, extend the fingers.

3. Bend your left arm at the elbow and bring it behind your back. Bring your palm to the right side and grab the big toe of your left foot with your hand. Help yourself by pulling your left shoulder back.

4. Try to move the knee of the left leg closer to the right leg. Stretch your right hand in your right foot and grab your foot with your palm.

5. While inhaling, stretch your back and look up.

6. As you exhale, bend your right arm at the elbow and tilt your body towards your right leg. Try to touch your knee with your forehead, nose, and chin. Keep your right knee off the floor.

7. Breathe freely. Count to 5. Slowly return to the starting position. Relax. Do the exercise on the other side.

If you cannot place the foot of one foot on the thigh of the other, then pull the heel of the bent leg as close to the groin as possible. Without reaching the big toe of the bent leg, stretch both hands forward, towards the foot of the straight leg.

The effect of asana on the body

This pose increases the flexibility of the knees and makes it easier to master the lotus position. Regular performance of this exercise relieves stoop and other posture disorders, and also improves blood circulation in the abdominal organs.

50. Triang mukhaikapada pashchimottanasana. Three-part forward bend pose

The word "trianga" means "three parts, limbs", this asana involves the buttocks, feet and knees. The name "Mukhaikapada" (touching the face of one leg) is formed by merging the three words "mukha" meaning "face", "eka" translated as "one", and "pada" - "foot, leg". Pashchimottanasana is a posture of intensive stretching of the back side of the body.

Asana technique

1. Sit on the floorstretch straight legs in front of you.
2. Bend your right leg and pull the foot outward toward your right buttock. Press the lower leg to the thigh, point the fingers back.
3. Shift your body weight to the right.
4. Stretch your arms forward and grab your left foot with your palms. Try to get your hands behind your left foot and grab your wrists with your fingers. Take two deep breaths in and out.
5. Press the knee of the right leg to the knee of the left. On exhalationtilt the body forward, bending and pushing the elbows. Try to touch the knee of the left leg with your face.
6. If you lose your balance, tilt your body slightly to the right.
7. Breathe freely. Count to 5. Slowly return to the starting position. Relax. Do the exercise on the other side.

The effect of asana on the body

Performing this exercise helps to get rid of flat feet and speed up recovery from sprains. Increased blood circulation in the abdominal organs eliminates violations of their work.

51. Crownchasana. Heron pose

The word "crunch" is translated as "heron".

Asana technique

1. Sit on the floorstretch straight legs in front of you.
2. Bend your right leg at the knee, pull it towards you, placing the foot at the hip joint with the heel up and toes back. Close your knees tightly. Take a deep breath.
3. As you exhale, bend your left leg at the knee, pull it towards you. Grab your left foot with your palms and straighten your arms and legs up. Straighten your back. Take 2 deep breaths and exhale.
4. As you exhale, move the body and head to the raised leg, trying to touch the knee with the chin. Make sure that the knee of the right leg does not come off the floor.
5. Breathe deeply. Count to 5. Slowly return to the starting position. Do the exercise with the other leg.

The effect of asana on the body

This asana effectively stretches the leg muscles and tones the abdominal organs.

52. Marichiasana I. Pose of Sage Marichi I

This asana got its name from the name of the sage Marichi, the son of Brahma and the grandfather of the Sun God Surya.

Asana technique

1. Sit on the floorstretch straight legs in front of you.
2. Bend your left leg at the knee and move your left foot towards you. Press the calf to the thigh, and the inside of the left foot to the inside of the right thigh.
3. Grasp your bent leg with your left hand, pressing the armpit against the outer surface of the left shin. Bend your left arm at the elbow, bringing your forearm behind your back.
4. Bend your right arm at the elbow and bring it behind your back. Grasp the wrist of the other with one hand, or interlace your fingers.
5. Turn the body to the left, look at the toes of the outstretched right foot. Take two deep breaths in and out.
6. As you exhale, tilt the body to the outstretched leg. Try to touch the knee of the right leg with your face.
7. Breathe calmly. Count to 5. Return to starting position. Relax. Do the exercise on the other side.

The effect of asana on the body

Strong contraction of the abdominal organs activates blood circulation in them and normalizes their work.

This exercise is useful for developing the mobility of the joints of the arm and increasing the flexibility of the spine.

53. Marichiasana II. Pose of Sage Marichi II

Asana technique

1. Sit on the floorstretch straight legs in front of you.

2. Bend your right leg at the knee and move under the buttocks. Point your fingers back.
3. Bend your left leg at the knee and move your left foot towards you. Press the calf to the thigh, and the inside of the left foot to the inside of the right thigh.

3. Grasp your bent leg with your left hand, pressing the armpit against the outer surface of the left shin. Bend your left arm at the elbow, bringing your forearm behind your back.
4. Bend your right arm at the elbow and bring it behind your back. Grasp the wrist of the other with one hand, or interlace your fingers.
5. Turn the body to the left, look at the toes of the outstretched right foot. Take two deep breaths in and out.
6. As you inhale, tilt your body forward, lowering your head to the knee of your right leg. Try to touch your knee with your chin.
7. Breathe freely. Count to 5. Slowly return to the starting position. Take a rest. Do the exercise on the other side.

The effect of asana on the body

This asana intensively heals the internal organs and significantly increases the flexibility and mobility of all joints.

54. Upavistha konasana. Sitting Angle Pose

The name of this asana is formed by the words "upavishtha", whattranslated as "sitting", and "kona", denoting "corner".

Asana technique

1.   Sit on the floorstretch straight legs in front of you.
2.   Spread your legs apart as wide as possible. Do not take your feet off the floor and do not bend at the knees.
3.   Grab your thumbsfeet in a pinch.
4.   Straighten your back, feel the ribs expand. Take 5 deep breaths in and out.
5.   As you exhale, tilt your body forward, trying to lower your chest and face to the floor. Pull your neck forward, touching the floor with your chin.
6.   Count to 5. Rise slowly, release your legs andrelax.
7.   Take a deep breath. As you exhale, lean to the left, grab your left foot with both hands and try to lie sideways on your outstretched left leg. Count to 5. Slowly straighten up. Relax. Do the exercise on the other side.

The effect of asana on the body

Performing this exercise is very effective for stretching the hamstrings and leg muscles. In this position, blood circulation in the pelvic organs improves and their health improves.

55. Pashchimottanasana (Ugrasana, Brahmacharyasana). Back and Buttocks Stretch Pose

The word "pashchimo", meaning "west", is usually used to name the entire back surface of the human body. The name of this asana translates as "Pose of intense stretching of the back of the body."

Asana technique

1. Sit on the floor, stretch your straight legs in front of you, put your hands on the floor near the pelvis with your palms. Take three deep breaths in and out.
2. As you exhale, stretch your arms forward, towards your toes, grabbing your big toes with your fingers.
3. Stretch your spine, arching your back slightly. Take three deep breaths in and out.
4. As you exhale, pushing your elbows apart, tilt your body forward, trying to touch your knees with your forehead.
5. Lower your elbows to the floor, touchingknees all over.
6. Wrap your palms around your feet. Count up to5.
7. Place your palms on the floor next to your feet. Count up to 5.
8. Slowly return to the starting position.

Master this exercise in stages - first achieve easy execution of the first stage of the asana, then the second, etc.

The effect of asana on the body

This asana has a tonic effect on the stomach, intestines and kidneys, improves digestion, activates the heart and heals the spine.

56. Parivrtta paschimottanasana. Reversed Back and Buttocks Stretch Pose

The word "Parivritta" is translated as "turned", Paschimottanasana - intensive stretching of the back side of the body. This asana is a variant of Paschimottanasana in which the body is twisted.

Asana technique

1. Sit on the floor, stretch your straight legs in front of you. Squeeze your legs tightly, tighten your knees.
2. As you exhale, stretch your left arm forward and reach for your right foot. Grasp the foot with the palm of your hand, pointing the little finger up and the thumb down. Take a deep breath.
3. As you exhale, raise your right hand to your left foot. Grasp the foot with the palm of your hand, pointing the little finger up and the thumb down. Take a deep breath.
4. As you exhale, rotate your torso to the right by 90°. Take a deep breath. As you exhale, move your head between your hands. Try to look up.
5. Try to get as low as you can, ideally touching your ribs to your thighs and bringing your left arm forward, touching your knee with your elbow.
6. Count to 5. Slowly return to the starting position. Do the exercise on the other side.

The effect of asana on the body

This asana is very beneficial for the spine and abdominal organs. This exercise relieves the feeling of fatigue and back pain, improves blood circulation in the pelvic area.

57. Urdhva Mukha Paschimottanasana I. Back Stretch Facing Up I

The combination of the words "urdhva mukha" is translated as "face up", Pashchimottanasana means intense stretching of the back surface of the body.

Asana technique

1. Sit on the floor, stretch straight aheadlegs.
2. Bend your kneesand pull your feet towards you.
3. Grasp your big toes with your fingers. As you exhale, straighten your legs together up. Try to fully extend your knees and arch your back. Maintain balance by sitting on your buttocks.
4. Try to move your hands so that your palms clasp your heels, or connect your hands behind your feet. As you exhale, pull the body and head to the legs, trying to touch the knees with the forehead. Pull your legs and spine up.

6. Count to 5. Slowly return to the starting position. Relax.

The effect of asana on the body

This exercise develops and stretches the muscles of the legs and back, improves posture and gait, and relieves fatigue.

58. Urdhva mukha pashchimottanasana II. Face Up Rear Body Stretch II

The name of this asana means "Intense stretching of the back of the body facing up."

Asana technique

1. Lie on the floor on your back, straighten your legs, tighten your knees, stretch your arms behind your head. Take two deep breaths in and out.
2. As you exhale, lift your straight legs off the floor and gently lift them up. Bring your legs behind your head, lifting your pelvis and lower back off the floor.
3. Grab your feet with your fingers. As you exhale, bend your elbows and spread them apart, pulling your toes to the floor. Try to touch your knees with your face.
4. Breathe freely. Count to 5. Slowly return to the starting position. Relax.

The effect of asana on the body

This asana is very useful for developing a sense of balance and coordination of movements. Intense impact on the muscles of the legs and thighs improves their shape.

Spinal traction relieves back pain and improves posture.

Regular performance of this exercise has a beneficial effect on the work of the abdominal organs, improves digestion.

59. Purvottanasana. Inverted Plank Eastern Stretch Pose

The word "purva" means "east" and is used to refer to the front side of the body. The word "uttana" is translated as "intense stretching".

Asana technique

1. Sit on the floor, stretch your straight legs in front of you. Place your palms near the buttocks, placing your fingers towards the feet.
2. Bend your knees, place your feet on the floor.
3. As you exhale, leaning on the feet and palms, tear off the body from the floor. Stretch your arms and legs, tighten your knees and elbows. Try to keep your body parallel to the floor. Stretch your neck, tilt your head.
4. Breathe freely. Count to 10. Slowly lower yourself to the floor. Relax.

The effect of asana on the body This asana is very useful for strengthening the ankles and wrists, it increases the mobility of the shoulder girdle, and expands the chest.

The word "purva" means "east" and is used to refer to the front side of the body.

60. Akarna dhanurasana. Archer Pose

The combination of the prefix "a" with the word "karna" ("ear") means "in the direction of the ear." Dhanurasana is the Bow Pose.

Asana technique

1. Sit on the floorstretch straight legs in front of you.
2. Stretch your arms forward and grab the big toe of the right foot with the fingers of the right hand, the big toe of the left foot with the fingers of the left hand.
3. As you exhale, bend your left arm at the elbow and the left leg at the knee, tear off the foot from the floor. Take a deep breath.
4. As you exhale, pull your left leg up, trying to bring your foot closer to your left ear. Do not bend your right leg at the knee and do not tear it off the floor.
5. Breathe freely. Count to 5. Slowly return to the starting position. Do the exercise with the other leg.

The effect of asana on the body

Regular performance of this exercise makes the muscles of the legs more flexible, the hip joints - mobile. This asana is very useful for normalizing bowel function.

61. Salamba Sarvangasana I. Candle Pose with Support I

The name of the asana is formed by the fusion of the words "sa" - "together" and "alamba" - "support, support", the resulting word "salamba" is translated as "leaning". "Sarvanga" is translated as "whole body". In general, this pose can be called "Supported asana for the whole body."

Asana technique

1. Lie on the floor, straighten your legs together, tighten your knees. Lay your hands along the body with palms on the floor. Breathe freely.
2. As you exhale, bend your knees and pull your hips towards your stomach. Take two breaths in and out.
3. As you exhale, lift your pelvis off the floor and place your palms on your lower back. Place your arms bent at the elbows on the floor with your shoulders. Take two breaths in and out.
4. As you exhale, stretch your torso up, using your palms to help it maintain a vertical position. The chin should touch the chest.
5. Move your palms to the middle of your back. Lean on the floor with the back of your head, neck, shoulders and upper arms. Take two breaths in and out.
6. As you exhale, straighten your legs, stretchingtoes up.
7. Breathe freely. Count to 5. Slowly return to the starting position. Relax.

The effect of asana on the body

This asana has a beneficial effect on the entire body as a whole, it is especially useful for normalizing the functioning of the thyroid and parathyroid glands. It is recommended for people suffering from shortness of breath, asthma, bronchitis, palpitations, frequent colds. The inverted position of the body and the free flow of venous blood normalize the functioning of the nervous system, relieve headaches, a tendency to increase pressure, insomnia and irritability.

Salamba Sarvangasana helps to establish normal bowel function and get rid of constipation.

This asana has a beneficial effect on the whole body. inin general

62. Halasana. Plow Pose

The name of this asana is translated as "Plow Pose".

Asana technique

1. Lie on the floor, straighten your legs together, tighten your knees. Lay your hands along the body with palms on the floor. Breathe freely.
2. Assume the position of Salamba Sarvangasana I.
3. Remove your palms from your back and place your outstretched arms behind your head, slightly lower your body to the floor.
4. Lower your straight legs behind your head and try to touch the floor with your toes.
5. Bending your knees, lift your torso.
6. Breathe freely. Count to 5. Slowly return to the starting position. Relax.

The effect of asana on the body

Regular performance of this exercise normalizes the work of all internal organs. Increased blood flow to the spine helps to get rid of back pain.

Improving intestinal motility relieves flatulence.

63. Karnapidasana. knees to ears

The name of this asana is formed by combining the two words "karna" -

"ear" and "pida" - "pressure", "inconvenience". Stage considered a continuation of Halasana (Plow Pose).

Asana technique

1. Lie on the floor on your back and perform Halasana (Plow Pose, p. 166).
2. Bend your knees, lowering them to the floor and moving your pelvis forward. The right knee should be located near the right ear, the left - near the left.
3. Stretch your toes. Try to connect your feet. Place your hands on your lower back or stretch them out.
4. Breathe freely. Count to 5. Slowly return to the starting position.

The effect of asana on the body

This pose has a beneficial effect on the whole body, allowing you to relax your legs, torso and heart at the same time. Stretching the spine significantly improves blood circulation in the lumbar region.

relax your legs, torso and heart at the same time.

64. Supta konasana. Recumbent Angle Pose

The name of the pose is derived from the words "supta", meaning

"to lie down", and "kona", which translates as "corner". This asana is considered one of the variations of Halasana (Plow Pose).

Asana technique

1. Lie on the floor on your back, perform Halasana (p. 166) and Karnapidasana (p. 168). Straighten your legs bent at the knees, spreading them as far as possible to the sides.
2. Pull the body up, moving the pelvis to your head, tighten your knees.
3. Grab your big toes with your palms, heels pointing up. Stretch your legs with your hands.
4. Breathe freely. Count to 5. Slowly return to the starting position.

The effect of asana on the body

The contraction of the abdominal organs that occurs in this position has a beneficial effect on their functioning. In addition, this asana has a tonic effect on the legs.

65. Parshva halasana. Plow Pose with Legs Behind Head

This variation of Halasana differs from the main version of the exercise by bending the torso to the side.

Asana technique

1. Lie on the floor on your back. Perform Halasana (p. 166).
2. Put your palms on your back a littleabove the waist.
3. Move the flattened straight legs to the right, supporting the torso with the palms. Do not move the body and chest, only the pelvis.
4. Breathe freely. Count to 5. Return to Halasana, move your feet to the left. Breathe freely. Count to 5. Slowly return to the starting position.

The effect of asana on the body

During the rotation of the spine, there is an active effect on the colon, which eliminates constipation and improves the passage of food through the gastrointestinal tract.

This pose is beneficial for developing the flexibility and mobility of the spine.

This variation of Halasana differs from the main version of the exercise by bending the torso to the side.

66. Eka pada sarvangasana. Candle Pose with One Leg Behind the Head

The word "eka" in the name of this pose is translated as "one", "pada" means "foot". When performing this asana, one foot is at the top and the other is on the floor.

Asana technique

1. Lie on the floor on your back and perform Salamba Sarvangasana I (p.

164).

2. As you exhale, lower your straight left leg towards your head. Try to put your toe on the floor without bending your knee. Make sure that the right leg is straight and extended vertically upwards.
3. Breathe freely. Count to 10. Slowly lift your left leg. Lower your right leg to the floor. Count to 10. Slowly return to the starting position.

The effect of asana on the body

This asana is extremely useful for normalizing the functioning of the kidneys and strengthening the muscles of the legs, abdomen and back.

67. Parshvaika pada sarvangasana. Candle Pose with One Leg Out to the Side

The word "parshva" is translated as "side". This pose is a variant of Eka Pada Sarvangasana, but the leg lowered to the floor is not located behind the head, but is retracted to the side.

Asana technique

1. Lie on the floor on your back, straighten your legs. Perform Sarvangasana (p. 164).
2. As you exhale, lower your straight right leg to the side. Don't bend your knees. Try to touch the floor with your toes.
3. Breathe freely. Count to 5. Slowly lift your leg. Perform the exercise with the other leg.

The effect of asana on the body

This asana is useful for strengthening the muscles of the abs and legs, as well as for the development of the hip joints. Also, this exercise has a beneficial effect on the functioning of the kidneys and intestinal motility.

68. Setu bandha sarvangasana (Uttana Mayurasana). Bridge Construction Pose

The phrase "setu bandha" is translated as "building a bridge."

Asana technique

1. Lie on the floor on your back. CompleteSalamba Sarvangasanu (p. 164).
2. Move your palms higher to your back, raise your body, bend your outstretched legs forward (in the direction opposite to your head) and bend at the knees.
3. Place your feet on the floor. The main weight of the body should be on the forearms, neck and back of the head.
4. Breathe freely. Count to 10. Slowly return to the starting position.

The effect of asana on the body

This exercise helps to get rid of tension in the cervical spine, relieves fatigue, and normalizes the functioning of the nervous system.

69. Setu bandhasana. Bridge Pose

The name of this asana is translated as "building a bridge."

Asana technique

1. Lie on the floor on your back. Take 3 deep breaths and exhale.
2. Bend your knees slightly, bringing your heels closer to your buttocks. Spread your knees, connect your heels.
3. Bend your elbows and place your palms on the floor on either side of your head. As you exhale, arch your spine, lifting your pelvis, hips, back, and shoulders off the floor. Rest your crown on the floor, moving your head closer to your feet. Cross your arms over your chest. Take 3 deep breaths and exhale.
4. As you exhale, arch your back, lifting your pelvis as high as possible, stretch your legs, straightening your knees.
5. Breathe freely. Count to 5. Slowly return to the starting position. Relax.

The effect of asana on the body

Performing this exercise is very beneficial for strengthening the muscles of the neck, legs and back and developing the flexibility of the spine.

70. Pindasana in Sarvangasana. Fetal Pose in Candle Pose

The word "pinda" is translated as "fruit", "embryo".

Asana technique

1. Lie on the floor on your back.Perform Sarvangasana (p. 164).
2. As you exhale, bend your right leg at the knee. Move the

foot of the right leg as close to the stomach as possible and place it on the top of the left thigh. Help yourself with your left hand. Take a breath.

3. As you exhale, bend your left leg at the knee, pull the foot towards you and place it on the top of your right thigh. Help yourself with your right hand.

4. Try to bring your knees as close as possible and stretch your legs up.

5. As you exhale, lower your legs towards your head. If the pose is easy for you, remove your hands from your back and wrap your arms around your crossed legs.

6. Breathe freely. Count to 5. Slowly return to the starting position.

The effect of asana on the body

This asana is extremely useful for normalizing the work of the digestive organs, it relieves flatulence and constipation. Also, this pose has a positive effect on the state of the thyroid and parathyroid glands.

Performing this exercise has a beneficial effect on the state of the nervous system, helps to relieve tension and calm down. Regular practice of this asana is useful for those who suffer from bronchopulmonary diseases, frequent colds and bronchial asthma.

71. Jathara parivartanasana. Belly Rotation Pose

The word "jathara" is translated as "stomach, stomach", and

"Parivartanasana" means "twisting", "turning".

Asana technique

1. Lie on the floor on your back. Stretch your arms out to the sides with your palms up.
2. As you exhale, lift your straight legs off the floor and lift them vertically up. Don't bend your knees. Take 3 inhales and exhales.
3. As you exhale, bend your legs to the right. Lower your legs towards the floor until your right foot is almost touching your right palm. Make sure your back and shoulders are completely on the floor. Keep your legs straight and tight at all times. If the left shoulder rises during movement, you should ask the assistant to hold it or put some heavy object on it.
4. Lowering your legs, move your stomach to the right.
5. Breathe freely. Count to 5. As you exhale, gently lift your legs vertically up.
6. Take three breaths in and out and lower your legs to the left. Breathe freely. Count to 5. Slowly raise your legs and return to the starting position. Relax.

The effect of asana on the body

This exercise actively tones the internal organs: stomach, liver, spleen, intestines, pancreas; helps in the treatment of gastritis.

Regular practice of this asana significantly reduces fat deposits in the waist and abdomen.

This posture is very useful for eliminating pinchings in the pelvic and lumbar regions.

72. Urdhva prasarita padasana. Pose of Stretched Up Feet

The name of this pose is formed by a combination of the words "urdhva", which means "from above, straight, high", "prasarita" - "lengthening, stretching" and "pada" - "foot".

Asana technique

1. Lie on the floor on your back, straighten your legs, tighten your knees, put your hands along the body, palms down.
2. Take a deep breath and exhale. Place your straight arms behind your head. Take two breaths in and out.
3. As you exhale, lift your straight legs off the floor and raise them 30 degrees. Count to 5. Take a deep breath.
4. As you exhale, raise your legs 60 degrees. Count to 5. Take a deep breath.
5. As you exhale, lift your legs vertically up. Count to 10. Breathe freely.
6. As you exhale, slowly return to the starting position. Relax.

The effect of asana on the body

This exercise strengthens the muscles of the legs, back and abs, and also helps to get rid of excess fat on the abdomen.

Regular performance of this asana normalizes the functioning of the abdominal organs, helps with flatulence and alleviates the condition with gastritis and colitis.

73. Chakrasana. Wheel Pose

The name of this asana is derived from the word "chakra", which translates as "wheel".

Asana technique

1. Lie on the floor on your back.
2. As you exhale, lift your legs off the floor, bring them behind your head, as when performing Halasana (p. 166). Take 3 deep breaths and exhale.
3. Bend your elbows and lower your palms to the floor near your head, placing your fingers in the opposite direction to the outstretched legs.
4. While inhaling, rest your palms on the floor, pull your legs forward and tear your neck and nape off the floor. Roll over your head.
5. Rely on your arms bent at the elbows, the crown and toes of your feet. Breathe freely. Count to 5. Smoothly roll back. Relax.

The effect of asana on the body

The rotation of the body increases the stretch of the spine and improves its blood supply. This asana is also useful for normalizing the functioning of all abdominal organs.

74. Supta padangushthasana. Stretching the leg for the big toe in the prone position

The name of this asana is formed by the combination of the words "supta", which means "lying position", "pada" - translated as "foot", and "angushtha" - "bigtoe".

Asana technique

1. Lie on the floor on your back, stretch your legs.
2. Bend your left leg at the knee and pull it towards your chest. Grasp the big toe of the left foot with the fingers of the left hand.
3. As you exhale, straighten your left leg straight up. Pull your leg closer to your head with your hand. Count up to 5.
4. Move your left palm to the popliteal fossa of your left leg, bending your straight leg towards you. Lift your head, neck, and shoulders off the floor and stretch your face toward your knee.
5. Count to 5. Slowly return to the starting position. Relax. Do the exercise with the other leg.

The effect of asana on the body

This exercise is useful for stretching the muscles of the legs and increasing the mobility of the hip joints.

75. Anantasana. Ananta's Serpent Back Pose

The name Anant in Indian mythology is called the god Vishnu and the serpent Sheshu, on whose back he sleeps.

Asana technique

1. Lie on the floor on your back. Take a deep breath. As you exhale, roll over to your left side.

2. Lift your head off the floor. Stretch your left arm, bend at the elbow and lower your head to the open palm.

3. Bend the right leg at the knee, clasp the big toe with the fingers of the right hand. Take 5 deep breaths in and out.

4. As you exhale, pull your right arm and leg up, extending your knee.

5. Breathe freely. Count to 5. Slowly return to the starting position. Do the exercise on the other side.

The effect of asana on the body

Active toning occurs in this pose hamstrings. This exercise is also good for the pelvic area.

76. Uttana padasana. Raise Arms and Legs Pose

The name of this asana is formed by the words "uttana" - "lying on the back, stretching" and "pada" - "leg".

Asana technique

1. Lie on the floor on your back. Connect your feet, tighten your knees. Take 4 deep breaths and exhale.

2. As you exhale, lift your back off the floor and bend it. Stretch your neck and, moving your head back, touch the top of your head to the floor (you can still rest your palms on the floor next to your head). Take 3 deep breaths and exhale.

3. Lift your tightly clenched legs off the floor and lift them up at a 45° angle.

4. Stretch your arms up and join your palms. Do not bend your knees and elbows.

5. Breathe freely. Count to 5. Slowly return to the starting position. Relax.

The effect of asana on the body

When performing this exercise, a complete expansion of the chest occurs, the flexibility and mobility of the spine increases, the muscles of the neck, back and press are strengthened. This asana is very useful for normalizing the functioning of the thyroid gland.

77. Bharadvajasana I. Pose of Bharadvaja I

This asana got its name in honor of Bharadwaja, the father of the famous commander Drona.

Asana technique

1. Sit on the floor, stretch your straight legs in front of you.

2. Bend the right leg at the knee, grab the foot with your hands and place it on the upper part of the left thigh, as close to the pelvis as possible.

3. Bend the left leg at the knee and take it back, placing the foot near the left buttock.

4. As you exhale, bend your right arm at the elbow, put it behind your back and wrap your palm around the toe of your right leg. Place your left hand on your right knee. Turn your body to the right, look ahead.

5. Breathe freely. Count to 5. Slowly return to the starting position. Relax. Do the exercise on the other side.

The effect of asana on the body

Performing this exercise is very useful for developing the mobility of the shoulder and knee joints.

78. Bharadvajasana II. Pose of Bharadwaja II

Asana technique

1. Sit on the floor, stretch your straight legs in front of you.

2. Bend the right leg at the knee, grab the foot with your hands and place it on the upper part of the left thigh, as close to the pelvis as possible.

3. Bend the left leg at the knee and take it back, placing the foot near the left buttock.

4. As you exhale, bend your right arm at the elbow, put it behind your back and wrap your palm around the toe of your right leg. Move your right hand over your right knee and lower your palm to the floor. Turn the body to the left, leaning slightly down and forward, look over the right shoulder.

5. Breathe freely. Count to 5. Slowly return to the starting position. Relax. Do the exercise on the other side.

The effect of asana on the body

Performing this exercise is very useful for developing the mobility of the shoulder and knee joints.

79. Marichiasana III. Pose of Sage Marichi III

Asana technique

1. Sit on the floorstretch straight legs in front of you.
2. Bend the left leg at the knee, place the foot on the floor as close to the buttock as possible. Press the lower leg to the thigh, the inside of the foot to the right thigh.
3. As you exhale, turn your body to the left, throw your right hand over your raised left knee.
4. Extend your right arm in front of your left leg. Take two deep breaths in and out.
5. As you exhale, bring your right forearm behind your left knee. Bend your right arm at the elbow and place your palm on your waist. Take a deep breath and exhale.
6. Put your left hand behind your back, bend it at the elbow. Clasp your hands behind your back. Turn your body as far to the left as possible. Turn your head to the right. Look over the right shoulder.
7. Tighten the outstretched leg, lifting the kneecap.
8. Breathe freely. Count to 5. Slowly return to the starting position. Relax. Do the exercise on the other side.

The effect of asana on the body

This exercise helps to get rid of pain in the back and hips, strengthens the muscles of the neck and increases their flexibility, develops the mobility of the shoulder joints. This asana is beneficial for the abdominal organs.

80. Marichiasana IV. Sage Marichi IV Pose

Asana technique

1. Sit on the floor. Pull outstraight legs in front of you.
2. Bend your right leg at the knee, pull your foot towards you and lower it onto your left thigh, as close to you as possible. Try to press the right heel to the navel.
3. Bend your left leg at the knee, place your foot on the floor and move your heel as close to your left buttock as possible.
4. As you exhale, turn your body to the left. Try to press the right armpit from the outside to the left thigh.
5. Bring the right shoulder behind the knee of the left leg. Stretch your right hand forward. Turn the body a little more to the left. Breathe in.
6. As you exhale, bend your right arm at the elbow and wrap it around the knee of your left leg. Lay the back of your hand on your back. Hold the left knee under the armpit of the right arm.
7. As you inhale, bring your left hand behind your back, with the palm of your left hand, clasp the palm or wrist of your right. Stretch your body up, turn your shoulders.
8. Breathe freely. Count to 5. Slowly return to the starting position. Relax. Do the exercise on the other side.

The effect of asana on the body

This exercise helps to get rid of pain in the back and hips, strengthens the muscles of the neck and increases their flexibility, develops the mobility of the shoulder joints. This asana is beneficial for the abdominal organs.

81. Ardha matsyendrasana I. Half pose of Matsyendra (Matsyendra - God of the Fish)

The word ardha means half. This asana is a light version of Paripurna Matsyendrasana - the Pose of the Fish God Matsyendra.

Asana technique

1. Sit on the floorstretch straight legs in front of you.
2. Bend your right leg at the knee, bring your right heel to your left buttock. The outer surface of the lower leg lies on the floor.
3. Bend the left leg at the knee, pull it towards you and move the foot over the right thigh. Lower your left foot to the floor on the outside of your right thigh or knee. The shin of the left leg should touch the right leg.
4. Rotate your body to the right and bring your right hand over your left thigh. Bend your right arm at the elbow, passing it under the left knee.
5. Bring your left hand behind your back, bend at the elbow. Clasp your fingers. Turn your head to the right. Look over the right shoulder.
6. Breathe freely. Count to 5. Slowly return to the starting position. Relax. Do the exercise on the other side.

The effect of asana on the body

Performing this exercise actively tones the lower abdomen.

82. Malasana I. Garland Pose I

The name of this asana is derived from the word "mala", which translates as "garland".

Asana technique

1. Stand on the floor with your feet together. Squat down without lifting your heels off the floor. Stretch your arms forward.
2. Spread your knees and hips to the sides, tilt the body forward so that the armpits touch the shins. Place your palms on the floor in front of you.
3. Put your hands behind your back and join your palms at waist level. Pull your back and neck up. Take 3 deep breaths and exhale. As you exhale, lower your head down, touching your forehead to the floor.
4. Breathe freely. Count to 10. Slowly return to the starting position.

The effect of asana on the body

This exercise is useful for strengthening the abdominal organs.

It is also recommended for girls during menstruation.

83. Malasana II. Garland Pose II

Asana technique

1. Stand on the floor with your feet together. Squat down without lifting your heels off the floor. Stretch your arms forward.
2. Spread your knees and hips to the sides, tilt the body forward so that the armpits touch the shins.
3. Put your hands behind your heels and join your palms. As you exhale, lower your head down, touching your forehead to the floor.
4. Breathe freely. Count to 10. Return slowly

The effect of asana on the body

This exercise is useful for strengthening the abdominal organs and getting rid of pain and fatigue in the back. It is also recommended for women during menstruation.

lower your head down, touching the floor with your forehead

84. Pashasana. loop pose

The name of this pose is derived from the word "pasha" - "rope",

"loop", because in this asana the arms wrap around the legs like a rope loop.

Asana technique

1. Squat down, keeping your heels off the floor. Bring your feet and knees together.
2. Rotate the housing to the left by 90°. Armpitthe right hand should be behind the left thigh at the level of the knee of the left leg. Bring your right knee forward 1.5-2 cm - this will improve twisting.
3. As you exhale, move your right hand in front of your left thigh, pressing

the armpit to the thigh, bend the elbow, the hand should touch the thigh. Take a deep breath in and out.

4. As you exhale, bring your left hand behind your back, bend at the elbow, bring the hand from the side of the right thigh and connect the hands.

5. Tighten your calves. Turn the body as much as possible to the left. Look left. Breathe freely. Count to 5. Slowly return to the starting position. Do the exercise on the other side.

The effect of asana on the body

This exercise is very useful for strengthening the calf muscles and developing ankle flexibility. In this asana, the legs get rest after standing for a long time. Twisting the spine increases its mobility.

In this asana, there is an expansion of the chest and the normalization of the work of the respiratory organs, a soft internal massage of the abdominal organs, and the resorption of fat deposits in the abdomen.

85. Kurmasana. Turtle Pose

The word "kurma" is translated as "tortoise".Turtle Kurma is one of the incarnations of the god Vishnu.

Asana technique

1. Sit on the floor, stretch your straight legs in front of you. Spread your legs 30-50 cm.

2. Bend your knees and pull them slightly towards you. As you exhale, tilt your body forward, bringing your right hand under your right

knee, your left hand under your left.
3. Stretch your arms to the sides, lower your shoulders to the floor. Take a deep breath and exhale. As you exhale, stretch forward, touching the floor with your face and chest.
4. Gently straighten your knees. The popliteal fossae should be near the armpits.
5. Breathe freely. Count to 5. Slowly return to the starting position or move into Supta Kurmasana.

The effect of asana on the body

This asana is considered an excellent remedy for balancing the mind and getting rid of nervousness.

Stretching the arms, legs, and spine in this pose actively tones the entire body.

The effect of asana on the body

This asana is considered an excellent remedy for balancing the mind and getting rid of nervousness.

Stretching the arms, legs, and spine in this pose actively tones the entire body.

86. Ardha matsindrasana II. Half pose of Matsyendra II

Asana technique

1. Sit on the floorstretch straight legs in front of you.

2. Bend your right leg and pull your foot towards you. Place your right foot on your left thigh as close to your stomach as possible.
3. As you exhale, bring your right hand behind your back, bend at the elbow, reach for the big toe of your right foot and grab it.
4. With your left hand, grab the big toe of your left leg extended forward. Slightly tilt the body forward, stretch the neck and lift the chin.
5. Breathe freely. Count to 10. Return to starting position. Do the exercise with the other leg.

The effect of asana on the body

This exercise is useful for increasing the mobility of the lower back and hip joints.

87. Supta kurmasana. Sleeping turtle pose

This asana is the final stage of Kurmasana, called the Sleeping Turtle Pose.

Asana technique

1. Take Kurmasana.
2. Turn your hands palms up and takethem back.
3. Bend your knees slightly, lifting them off the floor, slightly raise your chest. Bend your arms at the elbows and bring them behind your back. Connect the brushes at the level of the lower back. Pull your feet closer to your head.
4. Breathe freely. Count to 5. Slowly return to the starting position.

The effect of asana on the body

This asana is considered an excellent remedy for balancing the mind and getting rid of nervousness.

Stretching the arms, legs, and spine in this pose actively tones the entire body.

This asana is considered an excellent remedy for nervousness.

88. Vasishthasana. Sage Vasistha Pose

This asana got its name from the name of the great sage Vasistha.

Asana technique

1. Stand in Tadasana. Lean forward, rest your palms on the floor and move your legs 130-150 cm back.
2. Turn to the left, lifting your right hand off the floor. Lean on the left palm and the outer edge of the left foot. Press the right foot to the left, place the palm of the right hand on the right thigh.
3. As you exhale, bend your right leg at the knee, grab the big toe of your right foot with the fingers of your right hand. Straighten your arm and leg, stretching them up.
4. Breathe freely. Count to 5. Gently lower your arm and leg. Roll over to the other side and repeat the exercise with the other leg.

The effect of asana on the body

Performing this exercise is very useful for developing and strengthening the muscles of the legs, wrists, lower back and sacrum.

89. Bakasana. Crane Pose

The name of this asana is derived from the word "baka", which translates as "crane".

Asana technique

1. Squat down on the floor, connect your feet. Don't lift your heels off the floor.
2. Pushing your knees, lower your body forward. As you exhale, place your hands on the floor in front of your knees.
3. Bending your elbows, rise up on your toes. Leaning forward, place the shins with the front surface on the back of the shoulders (next to the armpits). Take 3 deep breaths and exhale.
4. As you exhale, shift your body weight forward and lift your legs off the floor. Hold the body in your arms. Look at the floor.
5. Breathe freely. Count to 5. Slowly return to the starting position.

The effect of asana on the body

Performing this exercise is very useful for improving blood circulation in the abdominal cavity, lumbar spine, sacrum and coccyx.

This asana well strengthens the muscles of the arms and shoulder girdle, contributes to the development of a sense of balance.

90. Eka pada galavasana. Pose of sage Galava with one leg

The word "Galava" is the name of an Indian sage. The combination "eka pada" is translated as "one leg".

Asana technique

1. Get on the floor on your knees. Gently tilt the body forward, lifting the pelvis off the floor. Lower your hands and head to the floor. Raise your pelvis and straighten your legs.
2. As you exhale, bend your right leg at the knee and place its foot on the top of your left thigh.
3. Tilt your body back until your legs are parallelsemi.
4. Bend your left leg, pulling it towards your body. Take 3 deep breaths and exhale. As you exhale, move your right foot over your left shoulder from the inside. Turn your toes towards your head. Place the knee of the right leg on the inner surface of the right shoulder. Take 3 deep breaths and exhale.
5. Straighten your left leg parallel to the floor. On exhalationlift the body, lifting your head off the floor, stretch your neck. Shoulders and forearms should form a right angle.
6. Breathe freely. Count to 5. Slowly return to the starting position. Do the exercise on the other side.

The effect of asana on the body

This asana is useful for strengthening the wrists and normalizing the functioning of the abdominal organs.

91. Supta bhekasana. Inverted Frog Pose

The name of this asana is derived from the words "supta", which means "to bow", and "bheka"- frog.

Asana technique

1. Sit on the floor, takeVirasana.
2. Turn your palms up andput them under your feet.
3. Pressing your hands on the feet up, tilt the body back. Take 3 deep breaths and exhale.
4. As you exhale, lift your pelvis off the floor, lower the top of your head to the floor, arch your back. Raise your feet so that your toes are on the same level with your pelvis.
5. Lean on your head, knees and elbows. The forearms should be at right angles to the floor.
6. Breathe freely. Count to 5. Slowly return to the starting position.

The effect of asana on the body

This posture has a pronounced tonic effect on the spine, improves its flexibility and mobility. This asana improves blood circulation in the neck, thighs, knees, legs, activates the work of the lungs and abdominal organs.

Pressing the palms on the foot strengthens the arch, which helps to get rid of flat feet.

92. Vamadevasana I. Pose of the sage Vamadeva I

The word "Vamadeva" is one of the names of Shiva.

Asana technique

1. Sit on the floor and take Baddha Konasana(Position of a shoemaker).
2. Place the palm of your right hand between the calf and thigh of your right leg. Raise the heel of your right foot, keeping your toes on the floor, and pull it towards your groin.
3. With your right hand, pull your heel towards the floor. Tear off the pelvis from the floor and lower it onto the right foot, press the knee to the floor.
4. Place the foot of the left foot on the right thigh, as close to the stomach as possible. Hold the left foot with the right hand.
5. Bring your left hand behind your back, bend at the elbow and bring the brush to the right of the body. Reach for your right wrist.
6. Turn your head to the right and look over your shoulder. Breathe freely. Count to 5. Slowly return to the starting position. Do the exercise on the other side.

The effect of asana on the body

This exercise is useful for developing the mobility of the leg joints. This asana improves blood circulation in the abdominal and pelvic organs. Twisting the spine heals it.

creator of the Indian language - Sanskrit

93. Hanumasana Monkey King Pose

The name of this pose is derived from the name of the strong and courageous leader of the monkeys Hanuman.

Asana technique

1. Kneel down on the floor, place your palms on the floor to the right and left of your feet.
2. Lift your knees off the floor. Move your left leg forward, right leg back.
3. As you exhale, try to stretch your legs as much as possible. Holding on to your hands, try to lower your pelvis as close to the floor as possible. Do not make sudden movements, master the pose gradually.

When you can fully lower yourself to the floor, place your hands in namaste.

4. Breathe freely. Count to 5. With your hands on the floor, raise your pelvis and switch legs.

The effect of asana on the body

This asana is very useful for the formation of a beautiful relief of the legs and the elimination of posture defects.

94. Samakonasana. Right Angle Pose

The name of this asana consists of the words "sama", which translates as

"straight, the same, similar", and "kona" - "angle". This pose is considered more difficult than Hanumasana.

Asana technique

1. Stand in Tadasana (p. 48). Put your palms on your belt and spread your legs to the sides as wide as possible.
2. Leaning your palms on the floor, as you exhale, lower your pelvis down, pushing your feet. As a result, you should be on the floor with your legs, the entire back surface and extended in one line, pressed to the floor.
3. Put your palms together in namaste. Breathe freely. Count to 5. Place your palms on the floor and slowly rise.

The effect of asana on the body

This exercise strengthens and stretches the muscles and joints of the legs, improves their shape, and increases the mobility of the hip joints.

Stretching the spine helps to form a beautiful posture, improves blood circulation in the pelvic area, and has a beneficial effect on the work of the reproductive organs.

95. Supta trivikramasana. Trivikrama Reclined Pose

The name of the asana is derived from a combination of one of the names of Vishnu - his dwarf incarnation - Trivikrama, and the word "supta", which means "to bow."

This is a rather difficult asana, it requires good stretching and long training. You should master it, feeling confident in Hanumasana.

Asana technique

1. Lie on the floor on your back, straighten your legs.
2. Lift your left leg off the floor and lift it up.
3. Stretch your arms and grab your heel with clasped hands.
4. As you exhale, pull your leg towards your head, making sure that your thumb touches the floor. Do not lift your right leg off the floor.
5. Breathe freely. Count to 5. Slowly return to the starting position. Do the exercise with the other leg.

The effect of asana on the body

Performing this exercise is very useful for stretching the muscles of the legs. This asana has a beneficial effect on the spine, preventing and eliminating problems with the intervertebral discs.

96. Urdhva Dhanurasana I. Inverted Bow Pose I

The word "urdhva" is translated as "up", so the name of this asana means "Upper Bow Pose".

Asana technique

1. Lie on the floor on your back.
2. Bend your elbows, place your palms on the floor behind your shoulders, fingers towards your feet.
3. Bend your knees and move your feet slightly closer to your hips.
4. As you exhale, lift your hips, pelvis and back off the floor, lean on your feet, palms and crown. Take 2 deep breaths and exhale.
5. As you exhale, lift your head off the floor, stretching your arms and legs and arching your back. Expanding the chest, bring up the pelvis.
6. Breathe freely. Count to 5. As you exhale, slowly return to the

starting position. Relax.

The effect of asana on the body

This exercise increases the flexibility of the spine and the mobility of the shoulder and hip joints. It is very useful for the formation of correct posture.

97. Eka pada urdhva dhanurasana. Reverse Bow Pose with Leg Raised

"Urdhva dhanurasa" translates as "Upper bow pose", a combination

"eka pada"means "one leg".

Asana technique

1. Stand in Urdhva Dhanurasana.
2. As you exhale, lift your straight left leg off the floor and lift it up as high as possible.
3. Count to 5. Lower your leg. Repeat the exercise with the other leg.

The effect of asana on the body

This asana is very useful for developing a sense of balance. anddeveloping good posture.

98. Kapotasana. pigeon pose

The name of the asana is derived from the word "bonnet"- "pigeon".

Asana technique

1. Sit on the floor on your knees. Spread your shins and feet apart and lower your buttocks to the floor between your heels. As you exhale, lower your back to the floor.
2. Stretch your arms behind your head. Bend your elbows and place your palms on the floor next to your ears, point your fingers towards your feet.
3. As you exhale, leaning on your palms, straighten your arms. Raise your torso, pelvis, and hips up. Try to bring your knees together.
4. Tighten your buttocks, arch your back. Bend your elbows and lower your forearms to the floor. Wrap your palms around your feet. Gradually move your head as close to your feet as possible.
5. Count to 5. Slowly lower yourself to the floor. Stretch your legs. Relax.

The effect of asana on the body

This pose increases blood flow.in the spine and pelvis.

Raising the diaphragm creates the effect of a gentle internal massage of the heart.

99. Dvi pada viparita dandasana. Reversed Staff Pose

The name of this asana consists of the phrase "dvi pada", which means "two legs". Viparita dandasana is the reverse, inverted Staff Pose.

Asana technique

1. Lie on the floor on your back.
2. Place your straight arms behind your head, bend them at the elbows, bring your palms under your shoulders, placing them with your fingers towards your legs.
3. Bend your knees. Place your feet on the floor close to your hips.
4. As you exhale, lift your body and pelvis off the floor and rest your crown on the floor. Take 3 deep breaths and exhale.
5. As you exhale, stretch your legs. Shift your body weight onto your neck, head, and arms.
6. Move the palm of your left hand behind your head. Place your forearm on the floor. Take 2 deep breaths and exhale. Move your right hand in the same way.
7. Tighten your legs, lift your pelvis as high as possible. Count to 5. Slowly return to the starting position. Relax.

The effect of asana on the body

This exercise makes the spine flexible and expands the chest.

This asana is very useful for people suffering from increased excitability.

100. rajakapotasana II. Pose of the King of Pigeons II

Asana technique

1. Sit on the floorstretch straight legs in front of you.
2. Bend your left leg at the knee, pull the heel as close to the groin as possible.
3. Take your right leg back.Place your palms on the floor.
4. As you exhale, bend your right leg at the knee, stretch your foot towards your head. Take 3 deep breaths and exhale.
5. Arch your back and tilt your head back. Raise your right arm above your head and bend it at the elbow. Grab the right foot with your right hand. Raise your left arm above your head and bend it at the elbow. Grab your right foot with your left hand. Try to bring your foot up to your head.
6. Count to 5. Slowly return to the starting position. Perform the exercise by changing legs.

The effect of asana on the body

This exercise is useful for all parts of the spine. It also strengthens and stretches the muscles of the neck and legs.

This asana does not improve the blood supply to the genital glands. andadrenal, thyroid and parathyroid glands.

101. rajakapotasana IV. Pose of the King of Pigeons IV

Asana technique

1. Get down on the floor on your knees, put your hands on the floor. Bring the left leg forward and the right leg back and straighten them (sit on

the twine - in Hanumasana).
2.   Straighten your shoulders, bringing your chest forward. Arch your back and tilt your head back.
3.   Bend your right leg at the knee and lift your foot up.
4.   As you exhale, take your right hand behind your head and grab your right foot with your palm. Take 2 deep breaths and exhale. Take your left hand behind your head and grab your right foot with your hand. Pull your foot towards your head.
5.   Count to 5. Slowly return to the starting position. Relax. Perform the exercise by changing legs.

The effect of asana on the body

This exercise is useful for all parts of the spine. It also strengthens and stretches the muscles of the neck and legs.

This asana does not improve the blood supply to the genital glands. andadrenal, thyroid and parathyroid glands.

102. Bhujangasana II. Snake Pose II

This asana is a variant of the Snake Pose.

Asana technique

1.   Lie on the floor on your stomach. Bend your elbows and place your palms on the floor at waist level.
2.   As you exhale, lift your head, shoulders, and body off the floor. Stretch your arms, bending your back, tilt your head back. Take 2 inhales and exhales.

3. As you exhale, bring your hands behind your back and place your palms on your legs as close to your knees as possible. Tighten your legs and buttocks, bend your back as much as possible back, without lifting your lower abdomen from the floor.
4. Count to 5. Slowly return to the starting position. Relax.

The effect of asana on the body

Performing this exercise is very useful for all parts of the spine. Stretching the muscles of the neck and shoulders increases their flexibility, relieves pain and fatigue.

Increased blood circulation in the abdominal cavity has a beneficial effect on the work of the adrenal glands and organs of the reproductive system. The work of the thyroid and parathyroid glands is normalized.

103. Rajakapotasana. Pose of the King of Pigeons

The word "rajakapota" is translated as "king of pigeons".

Asana technique

1. Lie on the floor on your stomach, stretch your legs. Bend your elbows and place your palms on the floor at your sides.
2. As you exhale, lift your head, shoulders, and body off the floor. Straighten your arms and arch your back. Take 3 deep breaths and exhale.
3. On the exhale, bendlegs at the knees, lifting the feet.
4. Arch your back, tilting your head back, trying touch the back of your head with your feet.

5. Breathe freely. Count to 5. Slowly return to the starting position.
Relax.

The effect of asana on the body

When performing this exercise, the blood supply to the pelvic organs is established, which contributes to the normal functioning of the genitourinary system.

This asana increases the mobility and flexibility of the spine and normalizes the functioning of the endocrine glands.

104. Padangushtha dhanurasana. Bow Pose with Thumb Grip

This pose is an intense version of Dhanurasana's Bow Pose. Its name is formed by the fusion of the words "pada", which means

"foot" andangushtha - big toe.

Asana technique

1. Lie on the floor on your stomach.
2. Bend your elbows and place your palms on the floor at chest level. Leaning on your palms, tear your head, shoulders and body off the floor.
3. Bend your knees and pull your feet towards your buttocks. As you exhale, bend your back, stretch your feet towards your head.
4. Place the foot of the right foot on the foot of the left. Leaning on the right hand, put your left hand behind your head and, as you exhale, clasp your toes with your palm. Take a deep breath.

5. As you exhale, lift your right hand off the floor and bring it behind your head. Grasp your toes with your right hand. Hold the left leg with the left hand, the right leg with the right. Pull your feet towards your shoulders.
6. As you exhale, stretch your arms and legs up. Count to 3. Slowly and carefully lower yourself to the floor. Relax.

The effect of asana on the body

Performing this exercise is very useful for maintaining the health of the spine and getting rid of slouching. Pressure on the abdominal aorta in this position activates blood flow in the abdominal organs, normalizing their work.

105. Gherandasana I. Pose of the sage Gheranda I

The name of this asnaah is derived from the name of the sage Gheranda.

This exercise connects you with Bhekasanui Padangushtha Dhanurasanu.

Asana technique

1. Lie on the floor on your stomach.
2. As you exhale, bend your right leg at the knee and pull your right foot to your right thigh.
3. Put your right hand behind your back and grab the foot of your right foot with your fingers. Take 3 deep breaths and exhale. As you exhale, press your hand on your leg, lowering it to the side and towards the floor.
4. Place your hand on the floor with your forearm in front of

you. Lift your head, shoulders and chest off the floor. Take 3 deep breaths and exhale.

5. Put your left hand behind your back, bend your left leg at the knee and pull your heel towards you. Grab your left big toe with your left hand.
6. As you exhale, stretch your arm and leg up. Tilt your head back, arch your back.
7. Breathe freely. Count to 5. Slowly return to the starting position. Relax. Do the exercise on the other side.

The effect of asana on the body

This asana strengthens and stretches the spine.joints of the hands and feet.

106. Natarajasana. Dance God Pose

The name of this pose consists of two words "nata", which means

"dancer", and "rage" - master. This asana is dedicated to Shiva, the God of dance.

Asana technique

1. Stand in Tadasana. Stretch your left hand forward.
2. Bend your right leg at the knee, lift it back. Grasp the foot of the right foot with the fingers of the right hand. Pull your leg back and up.
3. Try to bring your right thigh into a position parallel to the floor. The thigh and lower leg of the raised leg should form a right angle.
4. Bend your left arm at the elbow, turn your palm towards

you. Look at the fingertips of your left hand. Breathe freely. Count to 5. Slowly return to the starting position. Do the exercise with the other leg.

The effect of asana on the body

This asana is extremely useful for the formation of correct posture and the development of flexibility in the spine and joints of the legs. Regular performance of this exercise heals the kidneys and lungs.

107. Yoga mudrasana. Yoga print

Asana technique

1. Sit on the floor, stretch your straight legs in front of you. Take Padmasana (Lotus Pose). Perform Baddha Padmasana. Take a deep breath.
2. As you exhale, tilt your body forward, trying to touch your foreheadgender.
3. Count to 5. Slowly straighten up. Make byone slope to each knee.

The effect of asana on the body

When crossing the arms behind the back, a strong expansion of the chest occurs, which normalizes the functioning of the respiratory system. This exercise is very useful for developing the flexibility of the arms and legs.

This asana has a beneficial effect on intestinal motility.

Contents